THIRD OPINION

THIRD EDITION

AN INTERNATIONAL DIRECTORY TO ALTERNATIVE THERAPY CENTERS
FOR THE TREATMENT AND PREVENTION OF CANCER & OTHER DEGENERATIVE DISEASES

JOHN M. FINK

Avery Publishing Group
Garden City Park, New York

The publisher does not advocate the use of any particular form of health care but believes the information presented in this book should be available to the public. Treatments always involve some risk; therefore, the author and publisher disclaim responsibility for any ill effects or harmful consequences resulting from the use of any treatments listed in this book. The reader should feel free to consult a physician or other qualified health professional. It is a sign of wisdom, not cowardice, to seek an expert opinion.

Cover Design: William Gonzalez and Rudy Shur
In-House Editor: Jennifer L. Santo
Typesetting: Elaine V. McCaw and William Gonzalez
Printer: Paragon Press, Honesdale, PA

Avery Publishing Group
120 Old Broadway
Garden City Park, NY 11040
1-800-548-5757

Publisher's Cataloging-in-Publication

Fink, John M.
   Third opinion : an international directory to alternative
therapy centers for the treatment and prevention of cancer and
other degenerative diseases / John M. Fink. — 3rd ed.
   p. cm.
   Includes bibliographical references and index.
   ISBN 0-89529-770-1

   1. Cancer—Alternative treatment—Directories. 2. Alternative
medicine—Directories. I. Title.

   RC271.A62F56 1997

362.1'96994
QB197-40268

Printed in the United States of America

10 9 8 7 6 5 4 3 2 1

Contents

To Phoebe and Sharkey

Preface

My wife Sharkey and I had been married almost ten years before we felt we were ready to take on the responsibility of having a child. Phoebe, our little girl, brought us great light and happiness from the moment she was born. She was the best thing that ever happened to us, and when she was two and a half and doctors first diagnosed her as having a rare form of cancer, there wasn't anything we wouldn't have done to save her.

When the cancer recurred four months after a very difficult operation, and the conventional treatments of chemotherapy and radiation offered no hope (based on all previously recorded similar cases), we were willing to pursue anything that would offer a glimpse of hope as long as it wouldn't needlessly interfere with the quality of her life.

As Sharkey was seven months pregnant, we called our old Lamaze teacher to enroll in her class. Of course, we told her about Phoebe. She told me to call an actor that I'd been in a television series with and whom she had known through her classes. She said that he had been in similar circumstances with his mother about a year earlier and had turned to a complementary therapy.

I called him the next day, and he put us in touch with the Cancer Control Society, an organization in Los Angeles that provides information about unconventional therapies. They were very helpful in laying out some options among the alternative programs, telling us many of the things we needed to know to make a decision, and showing us how we could go about reaching various clinics, many of which were outside this country.

After numerous telephone calls, we chose a nutritional therapy for our daughter. Because we wanted the guidance of a doctor to help us get started, we went to a clinic in Mexico that specialized in this therapy under the auspices of Mexican doctors. There we were encouraged to undergo the therapy as a family to improve our health and prevent any health problems in our son, Andy, who had just been born.

Almost immediately after starting the program, Sharkey and I reaped health benefits. Sharkey's hay fever and chronic sinusitis cleared up completely, and she remains symptom free. My chronic hay fever and mild asthma, which had plagued me for twenty-three years and for which I, like Sharkey, had been receiving conventional treatment, went away. We began to believe in the relationship between diet and well-being. (In those days, the late 1970s, it wasn't even acknowledged by United States medical doctors that there was a link between most diseases and what you ate.) Our faith was reinforced at the clinic when we observed some patients with advanced cases of cancer, rheumatoid arthritis, diabetes, and heart disease responding well to the same diet.

Continuing with this comprehensive but demanding therapy over the next year and a half proved at times very stressful for us and our little daughter. After a few months, there were indications that the therapy on its own wasn't stopping the cancer. We tried introducing a few other harmless but potentially beneficial foods, herbs, and vitamins into Phoebe's diet. During this time we were greatly helped by all the information that came to us and by the assistance and support of others, who seemed to appear miraculously in times of need. Among them were people who showed us paths of healing in herbs, naturopathy, homeopathy, Eastern medicine, imagery, and meditation, just to mention a few. These people greatly enriched our lives.

In having taken the responsibility for Phoebe's well-being, we found ourselves learning to take responsibility for our own lives and, in doing so, tapping strengths and inner resources that serve us today. And during Phoebe's last months, we were very grateful to be able to help her to be free from the pain, suffering, and loneliness that often accompany cancer.

During the time Phoebe was still alive, we collected an enormous amount of information on complementary programs and talked with many recovered cancer patients. Piecing it all together wasn't easy. As our days were occupied in working on the therapy, we stayed awake late at night reading everything we could get our hands on concerning alternatives. Sharkey blazed the trails. She would read well after I had dropped off to sleep in exhaustion.

At some point in that year and a half, I had a vision of this directory. I knew that a guidebook would have been a tremendous help to us, and I knew that I would write it one day. Although I hadn't counted on its taking eight years from conceptualization to completion, I am convinced that there is a greater need than ever for this book.

I must pay tribute to Sue Carlan, who came as a college student to help me when I first rolled up my sleeves on this project. She spent hours and hours working on the various listings and showed courage where it failed me in fearlessly attacking my new computer and leading me gently along into this new technology. Her impish humor and high spirits equaled her dedication to and faith in this book, and I shall always be grateful to her.

After Sue left, James Rojas, already a wiz on the Macintosh, came to help. He showed me new ways of organizing the material and replaced Sue in working diligently on the listings in front of the electronic box. I am very appreciative.

My confidence in this project was greatly increased as a result of the time and commitment that Rudy Shur, managing editor of Avery Publishing Group, put into it. With Steven Blauer's input and good judgment, Rudy guided me toward better organizing and presenting this material. Additionally, editors Joanne Abrams and Laura Iacono of Avery kept throwing me the lifesaver. And Arthur Vidro was invaluable on the second edition, as were Karen Hay, Jennifer Lattanzio, and especially Jennifer Santo, on the third. I was lucky to find them all.

Deep appreciation goes to Sharkey for all her help and constructive comments. I couldn't have done this without her.

And no amount of thanks will do in crediting Michael Lerner for the time, encouragement, and support he showed for this undertaking since we first traveled together, looking at the clinics in 1982. His continual support of my work has meant a great deal to me.

For encouraging me to get a computer and do this book years ago, I am indebted to Stephan Schwartz, who was always there when I needed him and who spoon-fed me on the computer when I needed it. He also gave me many fine suggestions.

For reading the original manuscript and giving me many specific ways to improve this work, I thank John August, Grace Aldworth, Lorraine Rosenthal, Hal Card, Shirley Tyler, Jerry Freedman, and Dr. Walter Taylor.

For helping and heartening me, thanks to my other traveling companion, Dr. Sandra McLanahan, and to Ann Cinquina, Peter Barry Chowka, the late Marie Steinmeyer, Tom Atherton, Frank Wiewel, Chrystyne Jackson, Vivekan Flint, Larry Cooper, Beverly Seligson, Dan Beilin, and the late Betty Lee Morales.

For giving me guidance in getting a publisher, I owe a debt to Tom Monte, Ann Fransen, Hope Innes, and Ken Cohen.

To G. Haro, for having given me the Macintosh that made all this possible, "Muchimas gracias, Señor."

To the Reverend Jeffrey Duncan, Rabbi Wycoff, and Swami Satchidananda, for their inspiration, I am truly beholden.

Finally, to those who really deserve the ultimate accolades: thank you, Mother, for having put up with me all those years; thank you Sharkey, Andy, and Lily for putting up with me all these years; thank you, Phoebe, for having been such a wonderful teacher.

John M. Fink
Santa Barbara, California

Introduction

Third Opinion is strictly an information resource. Most of the progra⌁ ⌁⌁⌁⌁ed here are nutritional, metabolic, "immune enhancing," biological, or behavioral-psychological. Besides alternative therapy (given instead of conventional treatment) and adjunctive therapy (given with conventional treatment), they are often called complementary, unconventional, unorthodox, and nontoxic treatments. They are referred to by the American Cancer Society as unproven, although it has been pointed out that this is not the same as disproven. Many are considered holistic; they treat the whole body. They are relatively nontoxic—nondestructive to healthy cells. They often heal the body on many levels—mental, emotional, and spiritual, as well as physical. They often rely on a variety of substances, as opposed to a single substance, to stimulate the immune system and promote healing. (These multiple variables are one reason that current scientific standards are so hard to apply to these methods.) Moreover, these programs are usually aimed toward the cause of the disease and not just the symptoms.

The entire field of alternatives is vast and encompasses territory ranging from prayer to electromagnetic treatment. Although some may not be represented here, this book covers the majority of the better-known alternative therapies.

Doctors vary in their approaches to cancer. Patients commonly get second opinions, even several "second" opinions. However, rarely, especially in the United States, will a conventional doctor give you an enlightened opinion about nutrition and other non-toxic alternatives. For this reason, as well as the fact that there has been so little progress in healing the major cancers and other degenerative diseases, the interest in alternatives runs very high.

Although *Third Opinion* isn't for everyone, it may be for those of you who haven't found help in conventional treatments and are still looking and hoping. It could be for those who aren't ready to accept an "expert's" word as the final judgment ("you only have six months to a year to live"). It may also be for those people who want to assume responsibility for their own treatments, for those who are concerned about the quality of their lives, and for those who are looking for a gentler approach to healing in cancer, heart disease, arthritis, diabetes, multiple sclerosis, lupus, AIDS, or other degenerative diseases. And it could be for some of those patients who want to complement their con-

nts or reduce or eliminate the toxic side effects of those treatments.
his guide can and should serve those who are looking for ways to pre-
currence of cancer and other degenerative diseases. The diet-based pro-
e usually geared toward prevention. The importance of prevention cannot be
mphasized. Following the lead of the National Academy of Sciences' historic 1982
ort *Diet, Nutrition, and Cancer,* we can all begin by following the National Cancer
Institute's and American Cancer Society's dietary recommendations regarding fat
reduction along with an increase of fiber, including fresh fruits, vegetables, and whole-
grain breads and cereals. At the very least, we should be moderate with potentially
addictive substances such as alcohol, caffeine, sugar, and sodium. And it should go
without saying that we should stop smoking and limit our exposure to environmental
carcinogens: toxic substances and pollution. To all of this, add regular exercise. Among
the material here is much that can be useful in the field of prevention, for ourselves and
future generations.

I hope this book lists all of the nitty-gritty information about clinics, doctors, health
practitioners, educators, support programs, and research and information organizations. Because the field is so vast, it would take another book to present an in-depth
description and discussion of the therapies, underlying philosophies, supportive studies, case studies, and testimonials. For the same reason, I don't explore the historical,
political, or sociological aspects of alternatives. That kind of information can be gathered from the many books and articles listed in the bibliography and under the various
entries.

This book begins with guidelines that should be kept in mind as you consider the
various programs under discussion. The bulk of the book is divided into four sections:
Treatment Centers, which includes places where people can go for programs;
Educational Centers, which lists places where people can be educated about programs,
including some research institutes; Support Programs, which details programs giving
behavioral-psychological support, imagery training, and, in a few cases, material support; and Information Services, which explores organizations that specialize in information about all or some of the above and which lists patients' organizations as well.

As many approaches are somewhat eclectic, there is a certain amount of overlap in
some of these categories. Every section should be read to make sure that nothing of
value was skipped. To make it easier for readers to find resources in a certain geo-
graphical area, a region-by-region listing has been provided. Also included is a glossary of terms and abbreviations, and a bibliography. Telephone numbers given
throughout this book have been coded, whenever possible, to facilitate direct dialing
from the United States.

For some people, some of these methods may prove very difficult, both emotionally
and physically. The support of family, friends, and other helpers is very important. It
has been suggested that stress can slow down or even stop the healing process, so if the
necessary support isn't there or if something is contrary to your belief system, it might

be better to find a therapy you can participate in willingly and positively. Also, I fully support a person's choice to let go of the fight to survive whenever he or she feels that time has come.

It has been my dream over these past years to help bridge the gap between the worlds of conventional and alternative medicine. I believe that a patient is entitled to make an informed choice based on all the available information, and it is with this belief that I write this book. I urge you to keep an open mind about all therapies, whether they are conventional or unconventional. Each situation dictates a unique response. And I hope that considering these programs will not stop you from looking at conventional approaches, to use either alone or adjunctively, and pursuing them if they seem the most appropriate. Conventional programs, even the experimental ones, should be much easier to gather information about than those that follow, the difference being that conventional programs are sanctioned by the medical community while these are not.

Because the United States, unlike so many other countries, supports only one kind of medicine, Americans have overlooked many aspects of the art of healing. Economic, political, and professional pressures on institutional medicine have helped create an environment that deters the exploration of new avenues of research. This has made it very difficult for the health professionals outside of orthodox medicine to practice. It has also made it difficult for medical doctors to incorporate lesser-known healing methods into their practice. Because so many of them have been legislated against, harassed, prosecuted, and discredited, it is a wonder that so many of the champions of these therapies have managed to keep their programs available.

I must say a word here about quackery, as this, unfortunately, comes up so often. According to the late Congressman Claude Pepper's 1984 hearings on quackery, a quack is "anyone who promotes medical schemes or remedies known to be false, or which are unproven, for a profit." Now, of course, there are quacks out there who will try to take advantage of a cancer patient's situation for profit, both outside and inside mainstream medicine. And deceit, pretense, and fraud in serious medical matters are inexcusable and criminal. But it seems unfair to categorize unorthodox healing methods as quackery simply because they are "unproven." A United States government report* states, "it has been estimated that only 10 percent to 20 percent of all procedures currently used in medical practice have been shown to be efficacious by controlled trial." By this definition, wouldn't that make the remaining 80 percent to 90 percent of accepted medical procedures in the United States quackery?

I have seen many ethical practitioners using these therapies, helping people, working under duress, documenting their cases, and trying to get their programs recognized. It's a shame that all these practitioners can't get the attention of established medicine and receive funding for their research. However, the climate is slowly becoming more favorable.

Some United States congressmen took a step in the right direction when they

*Assessing the Efficacy and Safety of Medical Technologies, PB 286/929, Office of Technology Assessment, September 1978.

requested the congressional Office of Technology Assessment do a comprehensive report on *Unconventional Cancer Treatments.* This first government-sponsored look into these therapies, published in September 1990, cites many of the positive studies supporting these therapies while acknowledging the failure of orthodox treatments to make much more than minimal progress in bringing most cancers under control.

The report mentions the growing number of medical practitioners who choose to combine what they feel is the best of both alternative and conventional treatments, as well as noting how difficult it is to use unconventional methods in today's medical/legal climate. Stating that some of these methods may be adopted by mainstream practice in the years ahead, the report refers to recent progress in the psychosocial field, with the comment that many feel the next breakthroughs will occur in the nutritional area. It suggests the National Cancer Institute could take a more active part regarding unconventional treatments, such as by providing funds for conducting evaluations.

The relatively new Office of Alternative Medicine (OAM), which is part of the National Institutes of Health (NIH), is said to be, at least in part, an outgrowth of the report. Although their comparatively miniscule budget limits what they are able to do, the Office is beginning to selectively study what they believe are some of the more promising alternative approaches. Hopefully, outcome studies and other more practical and applicable studies will be increasingly valued, and the insistence on the grossly expensive, time-consuming, and impractical randomized clinical trials will diminish.

I continue to look forward to the day when most, if not all, of these therapies can be fairly assessed. In the meantime, before you undertake a program, the best means of precaution is to talk to people who've used it. The many patients who attribute their recoveries to alternative therapies will serve as a valuable source of help, inspiration, and information. Ask to talk to patients. Strong recommendations are a good defense against quackery.

You, the consumer, must be aware that there are people out there who will try to take advantage of your situation. The responsibility is yours to determine, through diligent research, who those people are, and then to avoid them. It is a fact that not everyone who tries a therapy, any therapy, is helped by it. It is also a fact that bad as well as good experiences occur with any therapy. To a large degree, your success will depend on when you go, who you see, and what you bring to that experience. Your attitude may be the factor that tips the scale toward good wherever you go.

Information can come to you in many ways, but you can't necessarily rely on an alternative doctor—just as you can't necessarily rely on an orthodox doctor—for all the information you may require. You are really on a solitary journey, and you should be encouraged to participate actively in your own recovery and perform your own research.

Everyone listed here was contacted by us and responded to our questions. If you cannot find a listing of the people or centers in which you're interested, we apologize.

In a few cases, people have asked not to be included, perhaps to avoid the kind of harassment often faced by professionals in this field. In some special cases, we decided that the reputation of a place was not good enough to justify its inclusion. However, it could be that we simply haven't heard of certain programs. If you will, send their names and addresses to Third Opinion, P.O. Box 50114, Santa Barbara, California 93150. We will get in touch with them before the next update.

There is a questionnaire for patients' comments in the very back of the book. Any feedback you can give us about your experience will be very useful and greatly appreciated. Just remove the questionnaire from the book, fill it in, and send it to the address on the form.

This book is an ongoing project. Since information becomes outdated as time passes, both the publisher and I are updating, revising, and reprinting *Third Opinion* to make it even more comprehensive.

I have not visited all the places listed in this directory, nor have I met all the practitioners. Although I have been involved with the International Association of Cancer Victors and Friends and with the National Health Federation, both information organizations, and have spoken before on this subject, it should not be construed that I am promoting or advocating any therapies or making recommendations of any kind. Nor should it be thought that I am assuming any responsibility for the decisions you may make. I am a layman passing on information for the reader to evaluate. A knowledgeable physician should be consulted regarding the medical aspects of any therapy.

It is my greatest hope that you will enjoy your search, that you will find what you need, and that your health will improve as a result of your efforts.

John Fink's Testimony Before the U.S. Senate Committee on Labor and Human Resources Hearing on "Nutrition and Fitness," Chaired by Senator Orrin Hatch, with Senator Edward Kennedy, Ranking Minority Member
November 13, 1985

I had been an actor for fourteen years when eight years ago, my two-year-old daughter was diagnosed as having a rare form of cancer. When doctors told us her prognosis was not good, my wife and I did what many loving parents do: we looked at anything and everything that could possibly help her. Our daughter lived only two years longer, but we feel that the quality of her short life was enhanced by the use of complementary treatments.

During our search we were surprised to find that many people with cancer were staying alive and well using natural methods. Some had advanced cancers and had been told by their doctors to go home and get their affairs in order. Many of these people are still alive today. This discovery consumed us.

For the past five years my wife and I have helped hold together a group in Santa Barbara called the Cancer Victors. Made up of around one hundred members, this group includes people with cancer, their families, and their friends. Those who have cancer are controlling it with nontoxic, primarily nutritional methods used exclusively or in conjunction with conventional treatments. Our work is volunteered and fills most of our time.

In 1982 I took several trips with professional researchers* visiting major hospitals, clinics, and physicians throughout the United States, Europe, and Mexico. During this trip I explored various complementary therapies and investigated the newest avenues of health research, prevention, and treatment of cancer and other degenerative diseases.

*Michael Lerner, Ph.D., who is a MacArthur Prize Fellow at the Institute for Health Policy Studies, University of California San Francisco School of Medicine. He is president and founder of Commonweal, a center for research in health and human ecology in Bolinas, California. Also, Dr. Sandra McLanahan, M.D., who is a physician from Charlottesville and Buckingham, Virginia.

I have brought two articles by Dr. Michael Lerner, one of the researchers. Published in *Advances,* the journal of the Institute for the Advancement of Health, these articles detail our findings and make them available for anyone interested.

In short, although we found no silver bullet cures, we found people who were reversing or at least holding their cancers in remission through the use of these therapies. As one example, we were very impressed with the Bristol Cancer Help Centre in England, officially opened by Prince Charles. The centre's program emphasizes a change of lifestyle, nutrition, and stress control, which often are added to conventional treatments to enhance the patients' response and powers of self-healing.

It made me sad to read Harvard statistician John Cairns' article, published in the November 1985 issue of *Scientific American,* in which Cairns said that of the more than 200,000 American patients receiving chemotherapy, the number of patients being cured could not exceed more than a few percent.

As Prince Charles said while addressing the British Medical Association: "It is frightening how dependent upon drugs we are all becoming and how easy it is for doctors to prescribe them as the universal panacea for all ills. Wonderful as many of them are, it should still be more widely stressed by doctors that the health of human beings is so often determined by their behaviour, their food, and the nature of their environment."

In our group in Santa Barbara, we see cancer patients coming back month after month who are keeping their cancer in remission by themselves using natural means. Many of them are aged. It often requires enormous determination, will, and courage to follow a rigid diet and do it alone, and their remissions seem anything but "spontaneous." What is tragic is that some of these people have to leave this country to find doctors who will or can monitor and support their progress while using these therapies.

I support groups such as the International Association of Cancer Victors and Friends and the National Health Federation* because, among other reasons, they are two of the few organizations supplying this difficult-to-get information about where people can go to find, for example, metabolic therapies, diet therapies, immune therapies, botanical therapies, and help in mental imagery. But this is not enough.

It is time that every doctor in this country recognizes the importance of nutrition and the mind, not only in preventing disease, but in helping to overcome

*These organizations were mentioned because of my association with them at the time. Please see information services for a complete listing.

disease. There is now a wealth of scientific information establishing the link between nutrition and the cause of some major forms of cancer. Clinical practice is showing us that nutrition can be an important complementary therapy.

Congress is to be commended for encouraging in the seventies the National Cancer Institute to set up the Diet, Nutrition, and Cancer Program, and for the creation of the Dietary Goals Report. Now the Congress, you Senators, can further the cause of improved health by calling for new research using nutrition in the treatment of cancer.

Thank you.

This study shows that many patients receiving alternative care do not conform to the traditional stereotype of poorly educated, terminally ill patients who have exhausted conventional treatment. Similarly, although some unorthodox practitioners may well fit the characteristic portrait of quacks and charlatans, many are well-trained, few charge high fees, and most, on the basis of patients' views and our own observations, sincerely believe in the efficacy and rationality of their work. Contemporary alternatives, unlike the pills and potions of the past, are long-term, lifestyle-oriented options that exist within a broad view of health and personal responsibility. Patients welcome the self-care role and the concomitant responsibility to attain health. . . . The emphasis of unorthodox therapy on nutrition, health as a personal responsibility, pollution, and purification has religious and moral overtones, but also represents themes of great importance not only to patients, but to science and society as well. As such, unorthodox therapy is unlikely to be readily discarded.

"Contemporary Unorthodox Treatments in Cancer Medicine"
Barrie Cassileth, Ph.D., et al.
Annals of Internal Medicine
July 1984

Half of the people interviewed said that clinics that treat cancer and other degenerative diseases in ways opposed by the established medical community should be allowed to operate in the United States.

Associated Press—Media General Poll
September 1-7, 1985

One in three respondents reported using at least one unconventional therapy in the past year.

"Unconventional Medicine in the United States"
David M. Eisenberg, M.D., et al.
New England Journal of Medicine
January 1993

Guidelines for Choosing a Therapy

The guidelines that follow should help in narrowing the choices presented here. Making decisions can be difficult. Even though the differences among the programs may be confusing, each one does not postulate a brand new principle. Look for the unity in the common underlying principles that are a part of so many of these approaches; they are often variations on the same theme. It helps to understand the concepts involved; if you don't already understand them, further reading may be essential. Examine each program carefully, but see it as a potential opportunity for getting well. Many of these guidelines can be applied to any therapy, whether mentioned in this book or not.

Similarities

A common denominator of many of the therapies is the idea that the body should rebuild itself through the use of fine nutrition, vitamins, minerals, and/or other "immune stimulators" that work as keys to activate the healing process. Some therapies emphasize that the body should first be detoxified through a cleansing process. Many of these theories are distantly related to the field of orthodox immunology but differ from most conventional treatments, which specifically target cancer cells but in the process can damage much more in the human organism.

These methods often deal with relatively harmless substances on the physical level, attitudinal changes on the psychological level, and the acknowledgment of some greater force on the spiritual level. They often are said to treat the cause, not just the symptoms.

Free Time

The more of this you have, the more options you may have. If you have to work full time, some treatments will be too time-consuming for you. Others, though, may be compatible with a busy schedule once you've begun. Some therapies are almost impossible to do without devoting your full time to them, at least initially. It is very important to recognize your limitations so that you don't commit to something unless you are in a position to follow through on it.

Belief Systems

If a particular therapy has some aspects that are going to add more stress to your life and you aren't able to curb your resistance, it may be best to look elsewhere. For example, I've seen a strict diet that is acceptable to one person be intolerable to another. (It's difficult to maintain belief in something you can't stomach.) Some programs built on a foundation of strong religious beliefs may not be suitable for someone who doesn't share those beliefs. I've seen meditation, as part of a program, conflict with a patient's religious convictions. There is a growing awareness that it makes a difference in what you have faith in, whether your faith is conscious or unconscious.

Comparisons and Statistics

Try to get information about people who have had a related cancer. Some information organizations, and some clinics as well, have lists of recovered patients who you can talk to. Call or write to these people, if you can, and ask what they specifically did that has helped them. Compare with conventional therapy results. These may be the most important questions you pursue, so spend some time on this.

With limited resources—no time, energy, or money—many alternative therapists find it impossible to compile statistics that would be acceptable to established medicine. And most of them simply don't have the capacity to do proper follow-ups. Again, you can ask for successful case studies. Unfortunately, statistics are questionable across the board—John Bailar of Harvard, in a 1986 study in the *New England Journal of Medicine*, and the government's 1987 General Accounting Office report both questioned the inflated conventional survival statistics stated by the National Cancer Institute.

Caveat emptor: Some doctors and clinics seem to be fond of concocting their own questionably high response and cure rates. Find out exactly what is meant by "response." Regard all cure and remission rates with some caution, and ask for documented cases and testimonials from clinics and doctors; sometimes you can get them.

Distance

A trip to another country might prove challenging and exotic to one person and debilitating to another. Language differences can be an obstacle, and clinics in other countries may not live up to what you have come to expect at home. Of course, they also may be just the tonic for you.

If you are unable for some reason to get to a center, then remember that some people have successfully undertaken programs at home.

Finances

You don't need the added stress of committing yourself to something that is financially over your head. There is a wide range of treatment costs, so think it through ahead of time. Take care to compare prices. You can do this most easily with centers that offer almost identical programs. Even though some prices may be outdated by the time you read this, if you consider the rough time frame in which they're current, they should form a good base for comparison. All prices are subject to change without notification, so check to confirm. Some programs will allow you to pay what you can afford. As many of these programs don't advertise this policy, you will need to ask specific questions.

Some therapies are covered by some insurance. This is a tricky area and always changing, so it's hard to give any hard-and-fast rules about how to handle this. Keep asking and trying.

Physical Condition

Your capacity for self-care and the extent of your illness will have a lot to do with your choice. Many therapies will take a lot of energy and might be next to impossible for some patients to accomplish on their own. For instance, obtaining supplies in bulk, growing certain foods, preparing particular diets and juices, and performing special procedures often requires the assistance of others. Sad to report, there is little active cooperation among the clinics, which means that if you are following a program that isn't working for you and you want to try a different program, you should not expect to be referred elsewhere. You will need both emotional and physical reserves to accomplish the move.

Clarity

Before you go to a clinic or an alternative practitioner, try to pin down exactly what you'll be getting and at what cost. That way you may avoid unwelcome surprises. Ask about patients you can talk to, find out about the length of stay and what you need to bring. Pin down what a practitioner means by "response" (get details on long- or short-term survival and ask questions about quality of life: lack of side effects, reduced or eliminated pain, enhanced well-being, etc.).

Some therapies have supportive studies to back them up; if not published in the United States, they are sometimes published in other countries. You can request to see them.

If you are going to another country and think there could be any confusion at all regarding arrangements, don't be afraid to check and recheck before you go. This is the best way to avoid unpleasant surprises.

Adjunctive Therapy

If it's important to you, when you contact a place ask whether the program can be used adjunctively as well as alternatively. The coordination of conventional and unconventional treatments could be crucial, so don't do this without good professional guidance. For example, if you are following a special diet on your own, be aware that it may not be compatible with chemotherapy. It's best to ask the right questions first.

Best Responders

If you are attracted to a center because of the responses you read under the listings, remember that these claims may be unverified; request that a place back up its claims by citing cases that you can verify. Some places did not specify which cancers have been most successfully treated by their program. Try to narrow it down to a type of cancer by specifying the cell type and stage of the cancer. If a place does not list a specific cancer, you should not assume that they are not having results with that type of cancer.

Be aware that all mentions of acquired immune deficiency syndrome (AIDS) are in response to a specific question we asked; we have no information to support the results.

Support

This is an extremely important area to consider; not only will the emotional support of your family and friends be important, but you may also need the physical support of someone to help you with the program. If support doesn't exist among those close to you, you may want to find people who are sympathetic and supportive. Support programs and information resource listings should be of great value in this area.

Verification and Consultation

This comprehensive list of people and places should in no way be understood to mean that either the author or the publisher recommends or endorses any of these therapies. The information was derived from questionnaires that were sent out and returned, along with other materials, and we did not make personal investigations into the accuracy of all the claims made here. Every patient should make his or her own investigation of the information on the list. In addition, it would be wise to consult with a knowledgeable physician before undertaking a therapy. Try to find a doctor who is sympathetic to your point of view. Obviously, this may take some time, but it will be worth the effort. A physician who listens with an open mind can be an invaluable source of support and guidance.

AFTER YOU CHOOSE A THERAPY

When you make a choice, do your very best to follow through. If you are bothered by the disorganization and confusion you might find at some centers, try to remain open and to give the program a fair trial. Do not abandon the program for reasons that may simply be conditioned prejudice. Beyond the surface, there may be much merit.

As with any therapy, close observation is important. Be alert to progress being made. Stay open to trying something different if what you're doing clearly isn't working or is working against you. Augmenting some therapies with parts of others may be okay, and by asking, you may find out about other people who have done this successfully; it may work for you, too. However, everyone is biochemically unique, so one person's needs may be different from another's.

The importance of your attitude cannot be overemphasized. Being confused over any period of time can only add to stress and may therefore impede the healing process. As mentioned earlier, when examining these choices, look for the unifying principle underlying most of them. See these choices as possibilities, opportunities, and gifts—which is what they are—and not as additional burdens. Believe it or not, I have often heard people say that getting cancer was the best thing that ever happened to them. By that they meant that with their backs to the wall, they finally found the motivation to examine and change their lifestyles and develop a strong will to live. On the subject of false hope, they say that there is no such thing.

TREATMENT CENTERS

Hospitals, Clinics, Physicians, Health Practitioners
North America (Bahamas, Canada, Cuba, Mexico, United States)

Accent on Health

2290 10th Avenue
Lake Worth, Florida 33461
United States

(407) 547-2770

7000 South Federal Highway
Stuart, Florida

(407) 220-1697

Contact Person

Mrs. Wallis.

Primary Personnel

Sherri W. Pinsley, D.O., medical director.

Directions

To Lake Worth: I-95 to 10th Avenue, west half a mile to a six-story building on the left called Concept Medical. Located in Suite 605. To Stuart: I-95 to Hope Sound, east to U.S. 1, then north to a three-story building.

Illness Treated

Breast, bone, prostate, lung, brain, and other cancers; chronic fatigue syndrome; immune suppressive diseases; candida; multiple sclerosis; Parkinson's disease; and chronic and acute pain.

Treatment Offered

Intravenous treatments including chelation, vitamins and minerals, and hydrogen peroxide; nutritional counseling; stress management; and lifestyle modifications. For pain: medications, OMT, nonsteroidal injections, and other therapies.

Related Readings

Books and articles from the American College of Alternative Medicine, American Academy of Pain Management, and Pain Society.

Length of Treatment/Stay

One to three months on average.

Costs

From $100 to $3,000 for three-month program, on average.

Method of Payment

Cash, checks, and credit cards are accepted. Insurance is accepted for some forms of treatment, but not for IVs.

Advanced Medical Clinic

17815 Ventura Boulevard, #113
Encino, California 91316
United States

(818) 345-8721
Fax: (818) 345-7150

Contact Person

Tracie Dario.

Primary Personnel

Ilona Abraham, M.D.

Directions

Take the Ventura Freeway, exit White Oak to South; turn right on Ventura Boulevard, go one-and-a-half blocks west to the clinic. Turn into street-level garage (parking is free), then take elevator to the first floor.

Background

The most important factor is to make a precise biological terrain diagnosis, and match it against dental or sinus foci. Then an appropriate immune system response is evoked by the individualized therapy.

Illness Treated

Chronic degenerative illnesses, including cancer, heavy metal toxicity (lead, mercury, cadmium), and chronic depression of the immune system.

Treatment Offered

Chelation therapy, total mercury detoxification, neural therapy, pain management, EAV (electrodermal skin testing), nutritional supplements and IV therapy, and natural hormone replacement therapy.

Related Readings

Toxic Metal Syndrome by Carsdorph and Walker.

The Care for All Cancers by Clark.
The Amino Revolution by Erdman.
Townsend Letter for Doctors and Patients by Collin.

Length of Treatment/Stay

Ambulatory—twice a week for six months.

Costs

Individual sessions, $200.

Method of Payment

Cash, checks, Visa, and MasterCard are accepted. Many services are covered by Medicare.

Advanced Medical Group

United States Office:
5862 Cromo Drive, Suite 147
El Paso, Texas 79912
United States

(915) 581-2273
(800) 863-7686
Fax: (915) 585-2274

Clinic:
Ave. Lopez Mateos #1281
Cd. Juarez, Mexico 32350

011-52-16-13-84-58

Contact Person

William D. "Bill" Carson, (407) 364-9815 Florida number and fax; (800) 278-1209.

Primary Personnel

Francisco R. Soto, M.D., medical director; Javier Sandoval, M.D., assistant medical director; Carlos Azcarate, M.D., director of gastrointestinal unit; Alejandro Llamas, M.D., laboratory and pathology director; Lucrecia Soto, general manager; W.D. "Bill" Carson, marketing.

Directions

Patients are met at El Paso International Airport, Greyhound bus terminal, or Amtrak station. However, if driving: South across Chamizal Bridge from El Paso on to Avenue of the Americas to Paseo Triunfo De La Republica, turn left to Ave. Lopez Mateos. Turn right to #1281 (nine-tenths of a mile). Clinic is at the corner of Ave. Lopez Mateos and De Mayo.

Background

Dr. Francisco R. Soto graduated from medical school in 1982, and completed his residency in general surgery in 1986. In 1985, Dr. Soto witnessed the results of chelation therapy on a friend, and in 1986, Dr. H. Ray Evers permitted Dr. Soto to visit him and learn about chelation. Dr. Soto became Dr. Evers' assistant, and later medical director of his clinic in El Paso/Cd. Juarez. In 1993, Dr. Soto presented the first objective data of the success using his protocols in the treatment of prostate and breast cancer. These protocols have been enhanced and have proven effective in other types of cancers.

Illness Treated

Arthritis, cancer, diabetes, heart disease, coronary artery disease, circulatory problems, *Candida albicans,* Epstein-Barr virus, chronic fatigue syndrome, and most chronic degenerative diseases.

Treatment Offered

Daily chelation therapy; ozone therapy via auto-hemotherapy; physical therapy; electrotherapy; colon hydrotherapy; pulsating magnetic field therapy; microwave stimulator; syncardon to improve venous return and arterial blood flow to the lower extremities; shark cartilage; Koch vaccine; laetrile (vitamin B_{17}); BCG (Bacillus Calmette-Guerin) for bladder, lung, and breast cancer; carbonylgrappen grouping for cancer; parabenzachinon for heart disease, arthritis, and others; rhodizonsaure for chronic fatigue syndrome, viral and yeast infections; live cell therapy; thymus therapy; DHEA; growth hormones; melatonin; and enzyme and nutritional therapy.

Length of Treatment/Stay

For full treatment program, three to four weeks are recommended. Special programs are available: live cell therapy, four days; thymus therapy, seven days; and a detoxification program, three to five days.

Costs

The basic program costs $3,100 per week for non-cancer, and $3,750 for cancer patients, due to special treatments. This includes transportation, hotel room, and meals at the hotel and clinic. The four-day live cell program, including laboratory tests, physical examination, colonics, room and board, and the live cells: $2,500. The thymus program, including tests, physical, room and board, and two thymus injections daily: $2,100.

Cost of the detoxification program will depend on the extent of the treatments and the number of days involved.

Method of Payment

Personal checks, traveler's checks, and cash, all in U.S. funds, are accepted. Payments are due in advance, and all financial arrangements should be made prior to coming to the clinic.

Vahagn Agbabian, D.O.

28 No. Saginaw Street, Suite 1105
Pontiac, Michigan 48342
United States

(810) 334-2424

Background

Dr. Agbabian is a staff member at Pontiac Osteopathic Hospital, Department of Internal Medicine, Pontiac, Michigan. He has been in practice for over thirty-five years.

Illness Treated

Internal medicine—cancer, some infectious diseases.

Treatment Offered

Dr. Agbabian doesn't take patients away from their regular doctor or oncologist, but instead offers complementary treatments, especially nutritional support.

Length of Treatment/Stay

Treatment is a complement to the patient's regular therapy, and continues for as long as necessary.

Costs

Initial consultation: $150. Follow-up: $60. Additional visits: $50 to $60. Patients can obtain most supplements from their health food store, or the doctor can supply them.

Method of Payment

Cash is accepted. Some insurance and Medicare coverage are accepted as well.

The Alivizatos Treatment—
Hospital American Biologics

Mailing Address:
P.O. Box 431880
San Ysidro, California 92143
United States

011-526-681-3171
Fax: (619) 428-2571

Coordinating Office:
190 E. Calle Primera, Suite 204
San Ysidro, California 92173

(800) 262-0212

Contact Person

Call the coordinating office. Coordinators are also available at: (800) 676-4714 or (800) 359-5106. Brochures and video sent free upon request.

Primary Personnel

Dr. Rodrigo Rodriguez, M.D., medical director. Five full-time M.D.s are available on staff at all times.

Directions

Cross the border into Tijuana, turn left on Revolucion Boulevard, which becomes Agua Caliente Boulevard. After about two miles, you will pass Caliente Racetrack, then in two blocks, the large Ley Department Store. Turn left across from the store onto Azucenas Avenue; the hospital is a half block off Agua Caliente Boulevard.

Background

American Biologics Hospital is a full-service, in- and outpatient, thirty-bed hospital. Five full-time doctors, registered nurses, full laboratory facilities, surgical facilities, and specialists are available in-house. Specializing in cancer and related problems, the hospital treats the whole person, mind, body, and spirit. The hospital also offers other treatments for cancer and related diseases.

Illness Treated

Cancer: sarcomas, pancreas, prostate, kidney, lung, breast, stomach, melanoma, leukemia, lupus, and, because the treatment will pass the brain-blood barrier, brain tumors. The treatment is also effective for diabetes and arthritis (including rheumatoid arthritis), emphysema, and chronic fatigue.

Treatment Offered

The Alivizatos treatment (researched and developed by Dr. Hariton Alivizatos) uses a formulation that is nontoxic to normal cells while effectively being toxic to abnormal cells. At the same time, the treatment regenerates, modulates, and enhances the immune system so the body can withstand abnormal influences. This is accomplished by administering a formulation consisting of elements found in isolated or uncombined form in a normal and healthy human body. These elements, when combined in the treatment, have significant therapeutic benefits. Since the ingredients are found in the human body, the resultant product is nontoxic, so patients experience none of the ill effects normally associated with chemotherapy or radiation therapy. The patient will normally experience reduced pain and increased appetite. The treatment pierces the protein and lipid layers of the cancer cells, opening the door to the infusion of those cells to effectively begin correction of the patient's metabolism. The resulting effect starves the cancer cells and enhances the condition of the healthy cells. The expected result is normally rapid remission and the eventual disappearance of the malignancy.

Length of Treatment/Stay

The treatment consists of a series of twenty intravenous injections on a daily basis, except Sundays. For heavy involvement in lupus and liver patients, an additional five to ten treatments are recommended. Some patients return yearly for ten to twelve booster treatments, to insure their continued good health.

Costs

The cost for the full twenty-treatment program is $3,450, which includes all doctor's visits, examinations, and blood tests on an outpatient basis, as well as breakfast daily for the patient and a companion. Patients normally stay at the International Motor Inn in San Ysidro, and are bused to the hospital. Room and meals for twenty-three days for the patient and a companion, approximately $1,700. Additional treatments are $150 each.

Method of Payment

Cash; cashier's, personal, and traveler's checks; and Visa are accepted. Most insurance companies will pay part or all of these costs, lab work, examinations, office visits, etc. HMOs and Medicare do not cover any of these services.

Alternative Medicine Associates

2416 Castillo Street, Suite C
Santa Barbara, California 93105
United States

(805) 569-8825
Fax: (805) 569-0580

Contact Person

Rodney R. Paragas, M.D.

Primary Personnel

Rodney R. Paragas. M.D.; Pei-Lun Zhang, M.D.; Robert I. Reynolds, Ph.D., N.D.

Directions

Take Highway 101 north or south, exit at Mission Street. If traveling northbound, turn right on Mission; if southbound, turn left. Turn left at Castillo Street. Go past Junipero Street half a block to 2416 Castillo. The driveway is on the right; parking is behind the building.

Background

Dr. Paragas has been a family practitioner since 1975, with a speciality in acupuncture and energetics since 1988. He formed Alternative Medicine Associates in 1994. The clinic offers integration of East and West medical philosophies utilizing complementary therapies to support the balance of body systems and the quality of life.

Illness Treated

Cancer, side effects of Western chemotherapy and radiation therapy, chronic degenerative diseases, chronic pain, arthritis, asthma, bowel disorders, cardiovascular disease, addictions, stress management, multiple sclerosis, Parkinson's disease, Alzheimer's disease, fibromyalgia, chronic fatigue syndrome, and other disorders.

Treatment Offered

Acupuncture, traditional Chinese herbal therapy, nutritional therapy, medical massage, acupressure, osteopathy, qi gong, homeopathy, Ayurveda, naturopathy, psychological counseling, and hypnosis.

Related Readings

Foundations of Chinese Medicine by Giovanni Maciocia.
The Web That Has No Weaver by Ted J. Kaptchuk.
Dragon Rises—Red Bird Flies: Psychology and Chinese Medicine by Leon Hammer, M.D.

Acupuncture Energetics, A Clinical Approach for Physicians by Joseph M. Helms.
Organon of Medicine by S. Hahnemann.

Length of Treatment/Stay

These forms of therapy are very individualized, so length of treatment will vary from case to case. An average might be one to three months, with follow-up appointments as necessary for health maintainence.

Costs

Office visit charges can vary from $50 to $100 per visit. Treatment charges can vary from $100 to $200 per visit. Herbs are extra, and vary from $25 to $100 per week, depending on the case.

Method of Payment

Cash, checks, Visa, and MasterCard are accepted. Most insurance can be billed and will generally reimburse, depending on the limitations and deductibles of the policy. The patient pays applicable co-payments and certifies financial responsibility in the case of insurance non-payment. No HMO coverage is accepted.

Alternative Medicine Center of Colorado

7601 E. Burning Tree Drive, Suite 100
Franktown, Colorado 80116
United States

(303) 688-1111
Fax: (303) 688-3706
Internet: www.naturesdoctors.com

796 E. Kiowa Avenue, Suite B
Elizabeth, Colorado 80107

8200 E. Belleview Avenue, Suite 205E
Centrum Medical Center
Englewood, Colorado 80111

Contact Person

Joy or Rhonda.

Primary Personnel

Reiner G. Kremer, D.C.

Directions

Located in the Denver Metro area.

Background

Dr. Kremer has been active in treating degenerative disease. He is a member of the American Academy of Anti-Aging Medicine.

Illness Treated

Cancer, multiple sclerosis, coronary vascular disease, arteriosclerosis, rheumatoid arthritis, and osteoarthritis.

Treatment Offered

Improvement and restoration of the body's defenses, immune status assessment, herbs, hydrazine sulfate, chondroitin sulfate, biologicals, therapeutic nutrition, adjunctive therapies, gastrointestinal cleansing, and detoxification.

Length of Treatment/Stay

Depends on health of individual, but generally two to five days. An appointment is required. This is an outpatient facility, so the patient will need to stay in a motel.

Costs

Initial evaluation and review of treatment records, between $300 and $1,000. Motel, $70 per night average.

Method of Payment

The center asks that the patient pay in full the first day. Personal checks, traveler's checks, money orders, Visa, and MasterCard are accepted. Insurance is accepted, but be sure to check with your insurance company first.

American Biologics-Mexico S.A. Medical Center

United States Information Office:
1180 Walnut Avenue
Chula Vista, California 92011
United States

(619) 429-8200
(800) 227-4458
(800) 227-4473
(all for admissions office)

Hospital/Medical Center:
#15 Azucenas Street
Tijuana, B.C.
Mexico

Contact Person

Michael L. Culbert, D. Sc.

Primary Personnel

Rodrigo Rodriguez, M.D., medical director; Robert Bradford, Ph.D. (Hon.), research director.

Directions

The hospital is located off Agua Caliente Boulevard.

Background

American Biologics-Mexico S.A. Medical Center, located in Tijuana, Mexico, is thirty-five minutes from the San Diego airport. This clinic has inpatient and outpatient care facilities. It offers a complete diagnostic laboratory screening, which includes standardized blood analysis, HLB and LBA blood monitoring, X-rays, CAT scan, and access, if necessary, to complete cobalt and other facilities. Standard orthodox therapies are available and integrated when jointly agreed upon by the medical staff and patient. Modern private and semiprivate rooms are available.

Illness Treated

Cancer and other degenerative illnesses.

Treatment Offered

Integrative, metabolic, nutrition, ACN bioelectricity, live cell therapy, tumor liquefaction, tumor blockers, butyrate complex and staphage-lysate in lymph system connected cancer, aqueous solutions of injectable laetrile, megavitamins/minerals, herbal non-surgical tumor removal, enzyme treatments, hydrazine sulfate, chondroitin sulfate, DMSO therapy, gerovital, experimental vaccines and biologicals, therapeutic nutrition tailored for the individual, sophisticated adjunctive therapies, EDTA chelation therapy (intravenous and oral), gastrointestinal tract cleansing, and detoxification.

Related Readings

Cancer Protocols by Robert Bradford and Michael Culbert.
Metabolic Management of Cancer by Robert Bradford and Michael Culbert.
Choice Magazine, sponsored by the Committee for Freedom of Choice in Medicine Inc.

What the Medical Establishment Won't Tell You That Could Save Your Life by Michael Culbert.

Now That You Have Cancer by Robert Bradford and Michael Culbert. Revised, 1991.

Oxidology: The Study of Reactive Oxygen Toxic Species (ROTS) and Their Metabolism in Health and Disease by Robert Bradford, Michael Culbert, and Henry W. Allen.

The Biochemical Basis of Live-Cell Therapy by Robert Bradford, Michael Culbert, and Henry W. Allen.

AIDS: Hope—Hoax—Hoopla by Michael Culbert.

Length of Treatment/Stay

Five days to three weeks.

Costs

Live cell therapy costs $2,700 for five days of treatment, including hotel. A ten-day total program costs $4,600. Live cell therapy injections alone are $200 per dosage. Degenerative conditions such as cancer, lupus, multiple sclerosis, emphysema, and others cost $2,000 outpatient or $3,600 for each week of hospitalization. A consultation visit may be arranged for $100. A diagnostic workup/consultation without treatment is $600.

Method of Payment

Most American insurance companies reimburse patients. Traveler's checks, certified checks, money orders, Visa, MasterCard, and American Express are accepted. No personal checks are accepted.

American Metabolic Institute
(Hospital Metabolico G. Rubio y Fry)

Mailing Address:
555 Saturn Boulevard, Building B, M/S 432
San Diego, California 92154
United States

(800) 388-1083
Fax: (619) 267-1109

Clinic:
Hospital Metabolico G. Rubio y Fry
St. Joseph Hospital
Calle Granados #420

Fracc La Mesa
Tijuana, B.C.
Mexico

(619) 267-1107
Internet: http://www.ami.health.com

(619) 229-3003
In Mexico: 011-52-66-21-76-02; 011-52-66-21-76-03; 011-52-66-21-76-04

Contact Person

William R. Fry.

Primary Personnel

William R. Fry, director; Geronimo Rubio, M.D., medical director; Kenneth Johnson, D.C., N.D., physiotherapy director; Gay Lynn Fry, counseling director.

Directions

The clinic is located three blocks from the Cinco y Diez corner in Fracc La Mesa, Tijuana, Mexico. Call for specific directions.

Background

The twelve-year-old clinic specializes in preventive medicine, and in treating degenerative diseases. Diagnostic tests include: blood crystallization test, live cell analysis, iridology, kinesiology, chiropractic, and traditional physicals, including: SMAC, CEA, CBC, urine blood panels, sonogram, CAT scan, MRI, and X-rays.

Illness Treated

Cancer, cardiovascular diseases, chronic fatigue syndrome, and other degenerative diseases, and preventive medicine.

Treatment Offered

Herbal salves on melanoma; detoxification program; fasting; colonic, colema, and enemas; bioelectrical medicine; hydrogen peroxide; laetrile; lymphatic massage; reflexology; clay baths; ultrasound; acupressure; hydrotherapy; chelation; growth hormone therapy; immunology; vitamins; minerals; amino acids; digestive enzymes; herbs; homeopathic remedies; vegetarian and metabolic nutrition program; colon therapy; magnetic therapy; ozone therapy; heavy metals, chemicals, and amalgam removal; attitudinal support with private counseling; group therapy; music relaxation and art therapy classes; and educational classes on nutrition and physiology.

Length of Treatment/Stay

Private room with telephone and twenty-four-hour doctor and nursing coverage is provided for all patients and their support person. The program is between one and five weeks, or longer. Cancer programs continue with home programs for approximately a year and a half, with monitoring done by the clinic. Outpatient programs are available.

Costs

Cancer program: $12,000 to $36,000 for three to five weeks. Candida/EBV program: Approximately $3,500 to $6,900 for two weeks. Chelation detoxification program: $6,000 for two weeks. Detoxification program: $1,700 for one week. Companions: $35 per day. Complimentary outpatient services, health screens consultations, and insurance processing services.

Method of Payment

Traveler's checks, money orders, Visa, MasterCard, and American Express are accepted. Most American insurance companies reimburse the patient. To check on insurance coverage, call (619) 267-1107.

Scott V. Anderson, M.D., D.C.

345 West Portal Avenue
San Francisco, California 94127
United States

(415) 566-1000

25 Mitchell Boulevard, Suite 8
San Rafael, California 94903
United States

(415) 472-2343

Contact Person

Lenore or Laura.

Illness Treated

A full range of chronic disorders, especially those that have eluded conventional care.

Treatment Offered

Nutrition, detoxification, herbs, IV therapies, all aimed at restoring function without resorting to pharmaceuticals.

Length of Treatment/Stay

Variable.

Costs

Variable.

Method of Payment

Cash is accepted. Some insurance is accepted; call to confirm.

The Ash Center for Comprehensive Medicine

800 A Fifth Avenue
New York, New York 10021-1216
United States

(212) 758-3200
Fax: (212) 249-3805

Contact Person

Janice Feldman, ext. 100.

Primary Personnel

Richard N. Ash, M.D., P.C., internal medicine.

Directions

Midtown Manhattan, 61st Street and 5th Avenue.

Background

The center offers alternative and preventative therapies for building and maintaining a strong, healthy immune system. It seeks to lower toxic load and replace vitamin and mineral deficiencies, and to get at the source of the problem rather than mask the symptoms.

Illness Treated

Cancer, HIV, chronic fatigue, allergies (environmental and food), depression, heart disease, arthritis, memory loss, and weight reduction.

Treatment Offered

Chelation therapy, oxidative therapy, reconstructive therapy (nonsurgical ligament and joint repair), vitamin therapy (oral and intravenous), and allergy treatments.

Length of Treatment/Stay

Varies according to the patient.

Costs

Initial consultation: $250. Other costs vary.

Method of Payment

Cash, checks, Visa, MasterCard, American Express, and Dencharge (credit card given by the office) are accepted. Insurance is not accepted.

Atkins Center for Complementary Medicine

152 East 55th Street
New York, New York 10022
United States

(212) 758-2110
Fax: (212) 754-4284

Contact Person

New patient representatives are Christine, Renee, and Binni.

Primary Personnel

Robert C. Atkins, M.D.; Stuart Fischer, M.D.

Directions

Located in midtown Manhattan, accessible by public transportation.

Background

Dr. Atkins has been in the forefront of the nutrition medicine movement ever since the publication of his book *Dr. Atkins' Diet Revolution.* He graduated from Cornell University Medical College, trained in cardiology, is president of the Foundation for the Advancement of Innovative Medicine, and is a member of the American College of Advancement in Medicine. He hosts "Design for Living," the longest-running health-related radio program in the United States.

Illness Treated

Cancer of all types, with especially favorable results for prostate and lung cancer. Also treats blood sugar disorders, chronic fatigue syndrome, autoimmune disorders, cardiovascular diseases, allergies, asthma, obesity, disturbances of lipid metabolism, and other chronic illnesses. The center prefers patients who have no prior exposure to chemotherapy or radiation.

Treatment Offered

Nutritionally based treatments, including oral vitamin and mineral therapy, dietary regulation, and an intensive intravenous program. Modalities include integrated protocols with herbal therapies, germanium, pancreatic enzymes, and oxygenating therapies.

Related Readings

Dr. Atkins' Health Revolution by Robert C. Atkins, M.D.

Dr. Atkins' Superenergy Diet by Robert C. Atkins, M.D.

Dr. Atkins' Nutrition Breakthrough by Robert C. Atkins, M.D.

Dr. Atkins' Diet Revolution by Robert C. Atkins, M.D.

Dr. Atkins' New Diet Revolution by Robert C. Atkins, M.D.

Dr. Atkins' New Diet Revolution Cookbook by Robert C. Atkins, M.D.

Length of Treatment/Stay

Intensive intravenous therapy requires frequent and periodic re-evaluations of blood parameters, of physical findings, and of standard procedures such as sonography and gastrointestinal scans. But there are no inpatient facilities; patients must make their own arrangements for housing.

Costs

Varies, depending on the type and extent of the illness and on the patient's response to treatment. An initial evaluation, on the average, costs $500 to $800. Additional costs—such as follow-up office visits, periodic laboratory evaluations, oral vitamin and mineral program, and intravenous therapy—not submitted for publication.

Method of Payment

No insurance is accepted. Patient is responsible for payment of services rendered.

Paul V. Beals, M.D.

9101 Cherry Lane
Laurel, Maryland 20708
United States

(301) 490-9911

2639 Connecticut Avenue N.W.
Suite 100C
Washington, D.C. 20008
United States

(202) 332-0370

Contact Person

Paul V. Beals, M.D.

Primary Personnel

Paul V. Beals, M.D.

Directions

I-95 or Baltimore-Washington Parkway to Route 198 to Laurel. To Route 197 South. Turn right at third light onto Cherry Lane. Office is on the left. The Washington, D.C. office is near the National Zoo.

Background

Dr. Beals is board certified in family practice. He is a certified clinical nutritionist, and has been practicing alternative medicine since 1981. He offers both conventional and alternative (complementary) medicine.

Illness Treated

All kinds of cancer; also heart disease, diabetes, chronic fatigue syndrome, fibromyalgia, lung disease, multiple sclerosis, vascular diseases, and all conventional diseases except AIDS.

Treatment Offered

Dietary and metabolic nutritional therapies, including IV and oral vitamins and minerals, DMSO, hydrogen peroxide IV therapy, BCG, chelation therapy, and others.

Related Readings

The Cancer Solution by Robert Willner, M.D., Ph.D.

Cancer and Nutrition by Charles Simone, M.D.
Bypassing Bypass by Elmer Cronton, M.D.
The Cancer Battle Plan by Elmer Cranton, M.D.
The Medical Miracle by Douglas Campbell, M.D.

Length of Treatment/Stay

For cancer: One to three times a week for three to six months. For chelation: One to three times a week for two to four months.

Costs

Cancer IVs: $75 to $95 each. Hydrogen peroxide IVs: $75 each. Chelation IVs: $95.

Method of Payment

Cash, checks, Visa, MasterCard, and American Express are accepted. Some insurance is accepted, including Medicare.

Daniel Beilin, O.M.D., L.Ac.

9057 Soquel Drive AB
Aptos, California 95003
United States

(408) 685-1125
Fax: (408) 685-1128
E-mail: dbeilin@got.net

Directions

From San Francisco, go south on 280 to 85 south, then to 17 south towards Santa Cruz. At Santa Cruz, continue south on Highway 1 to the Rio Del Mar exit and turn left, then left again on Soquel Drive.

Background

This outpatient clinic provides complementary therapies to standard oncology, and has established communications with oncologists who are open-minded to supplementary immune-system support. Dr. Beilin specializes in Sanum therapy, which provides a structural strategy toward correcting the body's own inner ecology, so as to actively decrease the possibility of a metastasis. On the patient's first visit, an initial homeopathic interview is provided, and the doctor utilizes darkfield microscopy, computerized thermography (a scanning method which examines the deeper areas of biological stress), and the Luscher test, which determines whether the illness has been influenced by the patient's ongoing psychological conflicts. He studies conventional laboratory findings, and orders new tests if he feels they could provide more sensitive and valuable information. He then designs a personal program based on the patient's individual history and needs, which is used with the orthodox treatment protocols the patient receives from his or her other physicians.

Illness Treated

Dr. Beilin treats the inner terrain of the whole system. He believes there is a surrounding reason for the tissue-related diagnosis, and he strives to find the real cause, rather than to treat the diseased tissue itself.

Treatment Offered

Enzyme therapy, diet, polypeptides, fungal cell-wall products, alkalinization, Chinese herbs, and correct thought.

Related Readings

Hidden Killers by Michael Sheehan, partial medical editing by Dr. Beilin.

The Body-Ecology Diet by Donna Gates. B.E.D. Publications.

The Substance of Homeopathy by Rajan Sankaran. Homeopathic Medical Publishers, Bombay.

The Cancer Microbe by Alan Cantwell, M.D.

The Challenge of Fate by Thorwald Dethlefsen. Coventure Press, London.

Paraclesus–Selected Writings edited by Jolande Jacobi. Bollingen Press, Princeton.

Mehr Heilungen von Krebs by Dr. Josef Issels. E. Schwabe Publishers.

Biological Transmutations by C. Louis Kervran. Happiness Press, 1987.

The Luscher Color Test by Prof. Max Luscher. Random House.

Cancer: Disease of the Soul by Dr. Geerd Hamer. Amici di Dirk, Publishers.

Length of Treatment/Stay

Therapy can begin on the first visit, pending urinalysis, darkfield, and thermographic results. Treatments are two or three days, with follow-up visits every three to eight weeks.

Costs

Approximately $250 per visit, including all supplementation. Total cost depends on length of treatment.

Method of Payment

Cash, personal checks, and credit cards are accepted. It is up to the patient to file for insurance.

Bio Medical Health Center

United States Clinic:
McCarran Quail Park
6490 S. McCarran Boulevard, Suite C-24
Reno, Nevada 89509-6118
United States

(702) 827-1444
Fax: (702) 827-2424

Philippines Clinic:
Bio Medical Health Center
2223 Marbella Building 1 #904 Roxas Boulevard
Pasay City Metro Manila
Philippines

Contact Person

Donna Webb.

Primary Personnel

David A. Edwards, M.D., H.M.D.; Corazon Ibarra Ilarina, H.M.D.

Background

Biological medicine, including homeopathy, acupuncture, bio-oxidation, chelation, herbal homotoxicology, nutrition, and neural therapy.

Illness Treated

Chronic degenerative diseases, vascular diseases, and heart diseases.

Treatment Offered

Anti-aging therapy, homeopathy, chelation, and traditional Chinese medicine. Please note that only the Philippines clinic provides treatment for cancer. The American clinic does *not* treat cancer.

Length of Treatment/Stay

Varies, depending on the condition being treated.

Costs

Varies, depending on the condition being treated.

Method of Payment

Cash, checks, Visa, and MasterCard are accepted.

Bio-Ethics Medical Center, Inc.

10752 North 78th Place #102
Scottsdale, Arizona 85260
United States

(602) 860-0490

Contact Person

Dr. Tano Lucero, president; Jennifer Weeter, office manager.

Primary Personnel

Dr. Tano Lucero, D.M.D., chemist, president; Dr. Todd Rhas, D.C.; Dr. Naida Brown, D.C.

Directions

Northeast corner of Pina and Shea, Scottsdale, Arizona.

Background

The center moved from Santa Fe, New Mexico, to Scottsdale in January 1993. It treats chemically-induced illnesses through detoxification.

Illness Treated

Cancer, chemically-induced illnesses, nervous disorders, allergies, skin disorders/hair loss, weight gain or loss, chronic fatigue, fibromyalgia, gastrointestinal disorders, headaches, mental confusion, depression, mood swings, and breast implants.

Treatment Offered

The center seeks to balance the body and open the energy pathways of the nervous, muscular, respiratory, skeletal, digestive, and lymphatic systems. Treatments rejuvenate and rebuild the organs of detoxification, such as the liver, gall bladder, kidneys, and colon. The center uses deep lymphatic drainage massage, electro-senscope (CNS balancing), acupuncture, herbs, supplements, nutrition, blood chemistry, homeopathy, chiropractic, and hair analysis.

Related Readings

Portraits of Homeopathic Medicines.
Recalled by Life by Anthony Sattilaro, M.D.

Length of Treatment/Stay

Most treatments are one hour long.

Costs

Therapies range from $35 to $50.

Method of Payment

Cash, checks, Visa, and MasterCard are accepted. The center accepts personal injury cases and preventive insurance coverage.

Bio-Medical Center

P.O. Box 727
3170 General Ferreira
Colonia Juarez
Tijuana, B.C.
Mexico

011-52-66-84-90-11
011-52-66-84-90-81
011-52-66-84-90-82
011-52-66-84-93-76
Fax: 011-52-66-84-97-44

Mailing Address:
Cristina Santos
P.O. Box 433654
San Ysidro, California 92143-3654
United States

Primary Personnel

Fernando Arriola, M.D.; Mildred Nelson, R.N.

Directions

The center prefers that the patient take the free shuttle bus from the International Motor Inn in San Ysidro; call (619) 428-4486. This insures that the patient is at the clinic before 9 a.m. The center does not take patients after 9 a.m.

Background

The Hoxsey therapy was started in 1840, when it was used on a horse with a cancerous sore on its leg. This formula was passed down through the Hoxsey family and has been used internally and externally on humans for more than fifty years. Mildred Nelson, R.N., now operates this clinic, which has been in Tijuana since 1963 and formerly was run by the late Harry Hoxsey. This is an outpatient clinic only. Appointments usually last one full day, sometimes up to three days, with a follow-up visit three to six months later, if possible. Patients are requested to arrive by 8:30 a.m. without having eaten breakfast and having taken a laxative the night before. Patients are given a complete workup in the morning, and meet with the doctors in the afternoon. Appointments are not necessary. The clinic is closed on all legal holidays of the United States; on five Mexican holidays—February 5, March 21, May 1, September 16, and November 20; and for the last two weeks of December.

Illness Treated

Most types of cancer.

Treatment Offered

Hoxsey herbal tonic and diet.

Related Readings

You Don't Have to Die by Harry M. Hoxsey. Joseph C. Carl, 1977. Available at the center or by mail; call for information.

Length of Treatment/Stay

One to three days as an outpatient.

Costs

Laboratory X-rays and physical examination charges run between $400 and $900. The charges must be covered on the day you are here. The Hoxsey treatment, for as long as necessary, is $3,500. A down payment of at least 30 percent toward the treatment must be paid on the first visit.

Method of Payment

Personal checks, traveler's checks, cashier's checks, international money orders, and cash in United States funds are accepted. No credit cards are accepted.

Block Medical Center

1800 Sherman Avenue
Evanston, Illinois 60201
United States

(847) 492-3040

Contact Person

The receptionists can answer all inquiries.

Primary Personnel

Keith I. Block, M.D., medical director; Mahmoud Mahafzah, M.D., Ph.D., oncologist; Charlotte Gyllenhaal, Ph.D., ethnobotanist, research associate; Mark Adjetey, Pharm.D., clinical pharmacologist; Dave Grotto, R.D., dietitian; Penny Block, B.A., director of education; Joseph Thomas, Ph.D., psychologist.

Directions

The center overlooks Oldberg Park and the campus of Northwestern University, and is within walking distance of Lake Michigan. It is easily reached via major thoroughfares and expressways, and is accessible from O'Hare Airport and the surrounding suburbs via public transportation and Metro train service. Visitor parking is available at no charge.

Background

Dr. Block's regimen was developed and studied over two decades and continues to undergo constant updating and revisions based on new scientific breakthroughs. His program includes the most up-to-date conventional medical treatments combined with unique and innovative strategies for battling and overcoming cancer. These are used in a deliberate, "gradualistic" fashion, with therapies and services adapted to each person's individual needs. This approach attacks illness and supports wellness from several directions at once, while identifying each patient's psychological, biomechanical, nutritional, and physiological resources to enhance well-being. Active involvement in treatment decisions and a meaningful partnership are at the core of patient care. The cornerstone of this center is a total approach to patient care, based on clinically sound experience and expertise, with its components solidly supported by the scientific literature.

The Block Medical Center is an outpatient facility, affiliated with local hospitals for necessary inpatient treatment. It provides total, comprehensive care for approximately half of all new patients. The others come for consultation and supplementary care.

Illness Treated

This program is designed to meet the varying needs of patients with a wide range of health concerns, from enhancing and maintaining good health to the treatment and prevention of serious illnesses, including cancer. The center's focus is on clinical care and research in strategies to improve cancer treatment, although other life-threatening illnesses are also addressed.

Treatment Offered

Meticulous medical workup with recommendations for procedures and treatments that boost immune, biologic, and emotional integrity; on-site conventional chemotherapy, when necessary, provided as "fractionated" therapy with innovative nutritional, botanical, and detoxification interventions to diminish side effects while enhancing therapeutic effectiveness; a therapeutic nutritional program tailored to the needs and food preferences of each patient; a fully developed plan of supplemental enhancers designed and recommended according to each patient's needs; stress management and relaxation techniques; psychological support service; cognitive training; private counseling; biofeedback training; massage therapy, including shiatsu, acupressure, and orthobionomy; electrotherapy, utilizing the electro-acuscope/myopulse system for chronic and severe pain without medications or invasive therapies; alternative pain management through a combination of biofeedback, myotherapy, acupuncture, and electrotherapy; prescriptive exercise; bio-conditioning; and health training.

Related Readings

Block, Keith I., M.D. "The Role of Self in Healthy Cancer Survivorship: A View from the Frontlines of Treating Cancer." *Advances,* Winter 1997.

Block, Keith I., M.D. "Complementary Approaches in Clinical Cancer Care." Presented at the annual meeting of the Association of Northern California Oncologists, June 10, 1995, San Francisco, California.

Block, Keith I., M.D., and Charlotte Gyllenhaal, Ph.D. "Emerging Progress in the War on Cancer." Presented at the Symposium on Adjuvant Nutrition in Cancer Treatment, March 17-19, 1994, San Diego, California. Published by Cancer Treatment Research Foundation, Arlington Heights, Illinois.

Block, Keith I., M.D., Charlotte Gyllenhaal, Ph.D., and Penny B. Block., M.A. "Dietary Change and Lifestyle Factors in Patients Surviving Advanced Malignancies." Presented at the Symposium on Adjuvant Nutrition in Cancer Treatment, March 17-19,

1994, San Diego, California. Published by Cancer Treatment Research Foundation, Arlington Heights, Illinois.

Block, Keith I., M.D. "Dietary Impact on Quality and Quantity of Life in Cancer Patients." Presented at the Symposium on Adjuvant Nutrition in Cancer Treatment, November 6-7, 1992, Tulsa, Oklahoma. Published by Cancer Treatment Research Foundation, Arlington Heights, Illinois.

Keith Block, M.D. "Integrating Diet, Fitness, and Psychological Support into an Oncology Practice." Chapter 17 of *Choices in Healing* by Michael Lerner, Ph.D., 1992.

Block, Keith I., M.D. and Charlotte Gyllenhaal, Ph.D. "Nutrition: An Essential Tool in Cancer Therapy." Office of Technology Assessment, Congress of the United States. *Unconventional Cancer Treatments* (OTA-H-405, U.S. Government Printing Office, 1990).

O'Connor, Amy. "A Nutritional War on Cancer." *Vegetarian Times,* May 1996.

Mead, Nathaniel. "Breakthroughs in Cancer Research." *Natural Health Magazine,* January-February, 1996.

Length of Treatment/Stay

Varies according to program selected. If a patient is seen on a consulting arrangement, a single visit may be scheduled. For those receiving ongoing care, the nature of the disease and/or the level of complexity of the case determines both the length and number of follow-up vists.

Costs

An initial visit costs $350 and includes consultation with an M.D., an R.D., and an R.N. Some scheduling can include a psychologist and a certified massage therapist. Subsequent visits are less costly than the initial consultation, and each ancillary service is then charged separately. A special discount is available in a nearby hotel for those staying several days. Laboratory fees are not included in the cost of the visit.

Method of Payment

Cash, checks, Visa, and MasterCard are accepted. Most commercial insurance is accepted. Most activities are reimbursable, except for some dietary and supplement interventions. Any questions should be referred to the office manager.

Brian E. Briggs, M.D.

718 6th Street S.W.
Minot, North Dakota 58701
United States

Office phone: (701) 838-6011
Reservations: (701) 852-1550

Contact Person

Dr. Briggs or secretary.

Primary Personnel

Brian E. Briggs, M.D.

Directions

Broadway to 11th Avenue S.W.; then four blocks west to 6th Street S.W.; then approximately four blocks north.

Background

Dr. Briggs is a 1954 graduate of the University of Minnesota (M.D.). He had orthodox experience in medicine and surgery before beginning holistic training and practice. The center's primary focus is on causative stress and environmental elements. The center takes three new patients per day and has twelve chelators.

Illness Treated

Cancer; the best responder is prostate. Also cardiovascular disorders, immune system disorders, psychological and chemical disorders, allergies, sensitivities, yeast, fungus, and mold infections.

Treatment Offered

Detoxification, elimination of environmental poisons, neural therapy, nutritional counseling, prescription drugs, and intravenous therapy of chelation and vitamins (with additional amygdalin in cancer patients).

Related Readings

Get Well—Stay Well (booklet for new patients), 1984.

Length of Treatment/Stay

One day to two weeks.

Costs

Lab (initial): $170. Office visit (initial): $150. Supplements: $100 (average).

Method of Payment

Cash and checks are accepted. Insurance is filed. Medicare covers only laboratory fees. Medicaid does not provide coverage.

W. Douglas Brodie, M.D.

309 Kirman Avenue #2
Reno, Nevada 89502
United States

(702) 324-7071
Fax: (702) 324-7639

Contact Person

Vicki Lowther, office manager.

Primary Personnel

Robert Kinney, R.N.; Livisa Valentine, clinical laboratory technician.

Directions

Located at the corner of Kirman and Ryland, near Washoe Medical Center. Take Highway 395 South from I-80 to Mill Street. Turn right on Mill (west) to Ryland. Turn right on Ryland to Kirman.

Background

Dr. Brodie provides immune enhancement for cancer patients, including specific substances that boost the immune system, such as thymus peptides, IV vitamin therapy, amygdalin, germanium, and other immune-enhancing minerals.

Illness Treated

All cancers. Best results are with lymphomas, melanomas, prostate cancer, and some cancers of the pancreas.

Treatment Offered

Megavitamin IV therapy, including amygdalin or laetrile, germanium, and ascorbate. Also used are carnivora, ukrain, hydrazine, butyrates, and azeloic acid.

Length of Treatment/Stay

Average, two to three weeks.

Costs

$1,500 per week. $4,500 to $5,000 for three weeks.

Method of Payment

Cash, checks, traveler's checks, Visa, and MasterCard are accepted. Insurance is accepted, but payment by insurance companies is not guaranteed. "Super bills" are given to patients to bill their insurance companies. Medicare is not accepted.

Buchholz Medical Group

1174 Castro Street, Suite 275
Mountain View, California 94040
United States

(415) 988-8011
Fax: (415) 988-8012
E-mail: drwnnb@pacbell.net

Primary Personnel

William M. Buchholz, M.D.; Susan W. Buchholz, Ph.D.

Directions

Follow Highway 280 and exit at Magdalena Avenue north. Cross Foothill Boulevard and street continues as Springer. Go one mile and turn right on Cuesta at the stop sign. Turn left on Miramonte at the light. Go six-tenths of a mile and enter complex from Miramonte just past intersection of Castro. From Highway 101, take 85 south. Follow signs to Grant Road/El Camino (Highway 82) north. Turn right on El Camino Real. Turn left onto Castro at light.

Background

Dr. William Buchholz is an oncologist who works with his wife, Susan, a clinical psychologist. They have been in practice since 1978. They offer a combined medical and psychological approach to cancer with an emphasis on integrating both conventional and complementary therapies. Dr. William Buchholz is a consultant to the Commonweal Cancer Help Program in Bolinas, California, and a cofounder of the Cancer Support and Education Center in Menlo Park, California.

Illness Treated

Cancer, hematology, and general medical problems.

Treatment Offered

Treatments include chemotherapy emphasizing the prevention of side effects, and control of symptoms from the illness and from treatment. Treatments are usually given in the office infusion center. Traditional Chinese medicine is available, including acupuncture and herbal medicine. Palliative and hospice care, including pain control, is also available. The group also provides consultation in complementary cancer treatments, and psychotherapy and counseling for individuals and families.

Related Readings

The Owner's Manual, A Guide for Owners of Human Bodies by William M. Buchholz, M.D., 1987.

Costs

A fee schedule is available.

Method of Payment

Insurance is accepted when services are covered. Otherwise, payment is expected at the time of service.

Burzynski Clinic

12000 Richmond Avenue
Houston, Texas 77082
United States

(713) 597-0111

Primary Personnel

S.R. Burzynski, M.D., Ph.D.

Directions

Directions will be sent along with prospective patient information.

Background

Dr. Burzynski treats patients with antineoplastons—nontoxic, naturally-occurring substances that "reprogram" cancer cells to die like normal cells.

Illness Treated

A wide variety of cancers. Best results have been observed with brain cancer, non-Hodgkins lymphoma, prostate cancer, and kidney cancer.

Treatment Offered

Antineoplastons, administered either intraveously or by capsule.

Related Readings

The Cancer Industry by Ralph Moss.

Length of Treatment/Stay

Varies widely, depending on patient response.

Costs

For intravenous therapy, approximately $5,000 per month.

Method of Payment

Cash, checks, and credit cards are accepted. The clinic provides patients with forms that facilitate filing with insurance carriers.

Cancer Treatment Centers of America

Midwestern Regional Medical Center:
2501 Emmaus Avenue
Zion, Illinois 60099
United States

Cancer Treatment Center of Tulsa:
2408 E. 81st Street
Tulsa, Oklahoma 74137
United States

Maryview Medical Center:
3636 High Street
Portsmouth, Virginia 23707
United States

(800) FOR-HELP

Contact Person

Oncology Information Services Department.

Background

Cancer Treatment Centers of America (CTCA) provides comprehensive inpatient and outpatient cancer care for both newly-diagnosed and later-stage cancer patients at hospitals throughout the United States.

Illness Treated

Cancer.

Treatment Offered

The CTCA treatment program combines traditional, research-based medical care—chemotherapy, radiation therapy, and surgery—with advanced treatments including autologous bone marrow transplantation, and several clinical research programs. Patients' treatment plans are supported by a nutrition program—diet planning, and vitamin and mineral supplementation—and psychosocial support—individual and family counseling, stress reduction, support groups, and relaxation programs, as well as mind-body medicine and pastoral or spiritual support.

Length of Treatment/Stay

Varies depending on patient need.

Method of Payment

Costs are covered by most commerical insurance companies, Medicare, and many managed care organizations (HMOs, PPOs, etc.).

Carolina Center for Bio-Oxidative Medicine

P.O. Box 32185
Raleigh, North Carolina 27622
United States

(919) 571-4391
(800) 473-9812
Fax: (919) 571-8968

4505 Fair Meadow Lane, Suite 111
Raleigh, North Carolina 27607
United States

Contact Person

Program consultant.

Primary Personnel

John Pitman, M.D., medical director; Wanda Arrendell, M.D.; Richard Salome, M.Ed., director of lifestyle and nutrition studies.

Directions

The center is located at the corner of Fair Meadow Lane and Atrium Drive in the Blue Ridge Plaza of West Raleigh, two blocks from Rex Hospital and the intersection of Lake Boone Trail and Blue Ridge Road. Take the Raleigh Beltline (I-440) to Lake Boone Trail toward Rex Hospital, across Blue Ridge Road to Atrium Drive (left turn).

Background

The center is an outpatient care facility that opened in October 1994. Initially, the center was established to offer an alternative to allopathic medicine in the treatment of immune system disorders (such as HIV, various cancers, hepatitis, chronic fatigue, and arthritis). This vision and practice have since expanded. Treatment programs now range from optimum wellness (sports medicine, family health counseling, and personal nutrition) to comprehensive health recovery (chronic immune system disorders, various cancers, digestive dysfunction, and cardiovascular ailments). Patients are housed in local guest suites and motels.

Illness Treated

All immune system dysfunctions, various cancers, and cardiovascular disease.

Treatment Offered

The three-week Bio-Oxidative Health Recovery program consists of daily treatments of ozone (various delivery methods), IV (EDTA chelation, vitamin C, hydrogen peroxide, minerals), modified diet with herbal detoxification, and hydrotherapy (colon or constitutional). Also included are complete medical evaluations, comprehensive laboratory testing and digestive analysis, lifestyle and nutritional counseling, and treatments in herbal body wraps and lymphatic massage. Other additional therapies may be suggested by the medical staff at an additional cost.

Related Readings

A Cancer Therapy by Max Gerson.
How to Reverse Immune Dysfunction by Mark Konlee.
Hydrogen Peroxide—Medical Miracle by William Campbell Douglass.
Juice Fasting and Detoxification by Steve Meyerowitz.
Oxygen Healing Therapies by Nathaniel Hawthorne.
The Chelation Way by Morton Walker.
Your Health, Your Choice by M. Ted Morter.

Length of Treatment/Stay

Minimum stay for cancer patients is three weeks in the Bio-Oxidative Health Recovery program. Recommended stay is four weeks.

Costs

From $10,500 for the three-week Bio-Oxidative Health Recovery program (includes all standard treatments and labs, weekly medical evaluations, education, food, standard supplements, and cost for housing).

Method of Payment

A deposit of 50 percent is required at the time of program reservation. An estimated balance is due on the first full day of treatment (usually Monday). Personal checks, certified checks, MasterCard, and Visa are accepted. Depending on the insurance contract, partial reimbursement is possible upon the client's submitting the proper forms to his or her insurance carrier.

Carolina Health Quest

1111 Quewhiffle Road
Aberdeen, North Carolina 28315
United States

(910) 281-5122

1009 N. Lake Park Boulevard
Box 16, Suite C-5
Carolina Beach, North Carolina 28428
United States

Contact Person

Tom Tripman.

Primary Personnel

Keith E. Johnson, M.D.

Illness Treated

ASCVD, CAD, PVD, arthiritis, COPD, CFIDS, cancer, and hormonal deficiencies.

Treatment Offered

Chelation, hydrogen peroxide, DMSO, ozone, hormone replacement, and colonics.

Length of Treatment/Stay

Twenty days. This is an outpatient facility, but the staff will help the patient find lodgings nearby.

Cost

$5,000 includes twenty injections, labs and blood work, and vitamins and supplements.

Method of Payment

$2,000 for drugs is paid directly to the pharmacist, and can be paid by credit card. The remainining $3,000 is paid by check to Carolina Health Quest. Insurance is not accepted.

Richard Casdorph, M.D.

1703 Termino Avenue #201
Long Beach, California 90804
United States

(310) 597-8716

Contact Person

Ms. Heidi Encz or Mrs. Joela Hayshida.

Primary Personnel

H.R. Casdorph, M.D., PhD., director of clinic.

Directions

Located in Long Beach, near 405 freeway.

Background

Graduate of Indiana University Medical School. Specialty training at the Mayo Clinic, Rochester, Minnesota. Ph.D. obtained from University of Minnesota. Diplomate: American Board of Internal Medicine, American Board of Chelation Therapy.

Illness Treated

General internal medicine problems with special interest in cardiovascular diseases, toxic metal exposure, and environmental medicine.

Treatment Offered

General internal medicine, EDTA chelation therapy, and nutritional medicine.

Length of Treatment/Stay

Varies with medical problem.

Costs

Varies with medical problem.

Method of Payment

Cash, check, or credit card is accepted at the time services are rendered.

Center for General Medicine and Acupuncture

(Centro de Medicina General y Acupuntura)

Avenue Ensenada #110
Tijuana, B.C.
Mexico

011-526-634-1412

Mailing Address:
P.O. Box 2757
Chula Vista, California 91912
United States

(800) 390-5610

Contact Person

Julian Mejia, M.D.

Primary Personnel

Julian Mejia, M.D.

Directions

The clinic is located in Tijuana, five minutes from the United States-Mexico border. After crossing the border, the clinic is at the corner of Ensenada Avenue and Boulevard Agua Caliente in Colonia Cacho, just five blocks from the Tijuana Tower Monument. Transportation is available.

Background

Dr. Mejia offers alternatives for the treatment of cancer and other degenerative diseases, incorporating various therapies while avoiding toxic side effects. He has worked with Dr. Harold Manner in establishing protocols using metabolic therapies. Emphasis is placed upon strengthening and improving the immune system. All treatment is available on an outpatient basis, and is based on the individual needs of the patient.

Illness Treated

Cancer, including brain tumors, breast cancer, colon cancer, lymphomas, lung cancer, and prostate cancer, as well as other types. Treatment is also offered for arthritis, osteoarthritis, multiple sclerosis, hypertension, osteoporosis, tendonitis, bursitis, chronic fatigue syndrome, and other degenerative diseases.

Treatments Offered

Complete body detoxification, diet and lifestyle changes, amygdalin (B_{17}), oral enzymes, immune therapy, chelation, and nutritional supplements for cancer patients. Acupressure and acupuncture for pain control as needed. Chelation and nutritional support is given to patients with various chronic degenerative diseases related to free radicals, circulatory system diseases, and calcium and cholesterol deposits within the different organs of the body. Colonics are offered on specific indications.

Related Readings

The Death of Cancer by Harold Manner. Advanced Century Publishing, 1978.

The Death of Cancer Update. Metabolic Research Foundation, 1988.

The Cancer Industry: The Classic Exposé on the Cancer Establishment by Ralph Moss. Paragon House, 1991.

Length of Treatment/Stay

For cancer therapy, eighteen days (Monday to Saturday). For chelation, six to twelve days, depending on the patient's condition.

Costs

Cancer therapy (eighteen days): $3,900. This includes all medical services, treatments, lab work, and diagnostic testing (X-rays, scans, ultrasound, pathology) as required. Chelation (twelve days): $1,200. This includes all medical services, full treatment, specialist consultations as needed, lab work, and X-rays. Local hotels in Tijuana will provide accommodations at commercial rates. Transportation from hotels in the United States to the clinic is available at no charge.

Method of Payment

Cash, cashier's checks, or traveler's checks are accepted. Insurance with pre-approval may be accepted with 60 percent advanced payment.

Center for Metabolic Disorders

P.O. Box 1134
Dania, Florida 33004
United States

(305) 929-4814

Primary Personnel

E.K. Schandl, Ph.D.

Directions

One mile west of Hollywood Beach on the Atlantic coast.

Background

The Center for Metabolic Disorders has developed a biochemical cancer profile done on a small vial of blood, which they claim can monitor the progress of cancer therapy and possibly foretell the development of malignancies more than two years prior to diagnosis. They use metabolic therapy as the main modality after preparation with vitamin C. Dr. Schandl also offers biochemical/nutritional consultations, which can be used to create metabolic programs for rehabilitation and improvement.

Illness Treated

Cancer, heart disease, multiple sclerosis, Parkinson's disease, viral and bacterial infections, lupus, malabsorption syndromes, AIDS, chronic fatigue, and candidiasis.

Treatment Offered

Metabolic-IV vitamin C, interferon, hyperbaric oxygen, colon therapy, physical therapy, nutritional therapy, and orthodox medical treatments, if necessary. For the CA profile, contact the laboratory for instructions on what to send and how to send it.

Length of Treatment/Stay

Tests are reported weekly.

Costs

Blood workup: $210 for the CA profile, plus DHEA-S and TSH. PTH for bone health, $90. Consultation: $210. Hospital fees, IV therapy, and other therapies all cost extra.

Method of Payment

For blood tests, only money orders are accepted. Insurance may cover approximately 80 percent of fees.

Center for Nutrition and Preventive Medicine

1355 15th Street, Suite 200
Fort Lee, New Jersey 07024
United States

(201) 585-9368

Contact Person

Lise.

Primary Personnel

Dr. Gary Klingsberg, D.O., medical director.

Directions

George Washington Bridge—upper level to Lemoine/Center Avenue exit. Proceed south on Lemoine to Main Street. Turn right on Main, and continue past first traffic light. Turn left onto Anderson Avenue. Continue on Anderson for approximately five blocks. Turn right onto Stillwell Avenue, then make a quick left onto 15th Street. Continue on 15th Street to #1355 (on right).

Background

The Center for Nutrition and Preventive Medicine operates under the premise that the combination of both medical and nutritional approaches to patient care is much more effective than either approach alone. Nutritional therapy is the treatment of choice, with the use of medications reduced or eliminated, so as to avert their unwanted side effects. While the use of drugs is important for the treatment of some disorders, the center prefers to address these problems through nutritional means where possible.

Illness Treated

Adjunctive therapies for breast, colon, prostate, and lung malignancies; cardiovascular diseases, including coronary artery disease and hypertension; endocrine disorders, including thyroid diseases and diabetes; arthritis; chronic fatigue syndrome; and environmental and food allergies.

Treatment Offered

Dietary and lifestyle modification; oral and intravenous vitamin, mineral, and herbal supplements; intravenous chelation therapy; osteopathic manipulation; and allergy treatments.

Length of Treatment/Stay

Varies, depending on the individual.

Costs

Varies, depending on the individual.

Method of Payment

Cash, check, Visa, and MasterCard are accepted. Participating insurance plans are accepted, and major medical plans are accepted once deductibles and copayments are met.

Center for Preve and Homeopathy

111 Bala Avenue
Bala Cynwyd, Pennsylvania 190(
United States

(610) 667-2927

Contact Person

Dr. Posner or Susan.

Primary Personnel

Howard Posner, M.D., medical di

Directions

From Route 76 (Schulkill Expressw
about one mile, turn right on Bala
from Route 1 south, Bala Avenue i
(Lancaster Avenue). The center is o... ... second block on the right side of the street.

Background

Dr. Posner has been practicing holistic medicine for over twenty years.

Illness Treated

Cancer, heart disease, arthritis, chronic fatigue, headaches, candida, hypertension, cholesterol, acne, infertility, and depression.

Treatment Offered

Treatments include megavitamins, herbs, homeopathic remedies, ayurveda, cleansing and detoxification, shark cartilage, and others.

Related Readings

Love, Medicine, and Miracles by Bernie Siegel.
Anatomy of an Illness by Norman Cousins.
Book of God's Love.

Length of Treatment/Stay

Long-term.

Costs
Average, $350.

Method of Payment
Cash, checks, Visa, and Ma
Personal Choice insuranc

60

sterCard are accepted. The center accepts Medicare and
e, and submits all others to help patients get reimbursed.

---

enters for Progressive Medicine

beck Health Center:
8 Montgomery Street
Rhinebeck, New York 12572
United States

(914) 876-7082

Center for Progressive Medicine:
Pinnacle Place, Suite 210
10 McKown Road
Albany, New York 12203
United States

(518) 435-0082

Primary Personnel

Kenneth Bock, M.D.; Steven Bock, M.D.

Directions

From the Taconic Parkway: Take exit for Rhinebeck—Route 199. Follow Route 199 West to Route 308. Follow Route 308 to Rhinebeck traffic signal; make a right onto Route 9 North. Take Route 9 North for approximately a quarter of a mile. As Route 9 bears to the right, continue straight ahead onto Montgomery Street. You will see the sign for Northern Dutchess Hospital. Go one-and-a-half blocks on Montgomery Street. The Health Center is on the left, in a large white Victorian house with blue trim. From points west: Take Route 199 East across bridge to Route 9G. Turn right on 9G East. Go approximately two miles to Route 9 South, and turn right. Go approximately two miles, and look for Northern Dutchess Hospital on the right. Immediately after the hospital, turn right onto Montgomery Street. Go one-and-a-half blocks; the Health Center is on the left.

Background

The center's personalized service is designed to satisfy and reflect the patient's unique needs, limitations, and expectations. Patients receive a comprehensive evaluation, which includes a complete medical history and physical examination, and a variety of individualized and specialized tests and diagnostic services. The result of this comprehensive evaluation is an individualized treatment plan.

Illness Treated

All types of cancer; food and inhalant allergies; chemical sensitivity; hyperactivity; attention deficit disorder; digestive disorders; chronic fatigue syndrome; autoimmune disorders; chronic viral infections; candidiasis; angina and other heart disorders; Lyme disease; premenstrual syndrome; osteoporosis; and menopause.

Treatment Offered

Adjunctive approaches to cancer; chelation therapy; dietary modification; herbal and Chinese remedies; enzyme potentiated desensitization; homeopathic medicine; photo-oxidation; oxidative medicine; and many others.

Related Readings

Bypassing Bypass by Cranton.
Into the Light by Campbell Douglass

Length of Treatment/Stay

Depends on type and severity of illness.

Costs

IV's: $85 to $100; chelation: $100; oxidative medicine: $100; photo-oxidation: $150.

Method of Payment

Cash, checks, Visa, and MasterCard are accepted. No new patients are accepted with MVP coverage; Medicare covers lab services only.

Central Coast Holistic Medical Services

32 East Sola Street
Santa Barbara, California 93101
United States

(805) 568-5594
(805) 899-4944

Contact Person

Jordan Goetz, M.D.

Primary Personnel

Jordan Goetz, M.D., medical director.

Directions

Route 101—exit Camillo Street. Go east one-and-a-half miles to Santa Barbara Street. Turn left and go up four streets to Sola Street. Turn left and go over one block to #32. Parking is in rear.

Background

Offers an integrative approach to medicine: a physician with training as a traditional M.D. and additional specialized training in alternative and complementary therapies. Treatment is unique for each client based on his or her needs.

Illness Treated

All illnessness are treated. Specialities include cancer, diabetes, and low back pain.

Treatment Offered

Primary care—coordinates and supervises all modalities of therapy. Physician skilled in herbal medicine, supplementation, and therapy with a holistic/whole person flavor.

Related Readings

Nutrition and Healing by Alan Gaby, M.D.
You Can Heal Your Life by Lonnie Hay.
Nutritional Influences on Illness.
And the writings of Bernie Siegel.

Length of Treatment/Stay

Ongoing, even when a "health challenge" has been overcome. Prevention is as important as treatment.

Costs

Based on level of service provided, from $45 to $100.

Method of Payment

Cash or checks are accepted. Payment is accepted at the time of the visit. The clinic has a billing service and will accept Medicare, but not on assignment.

Centro Profesional Unidad de Neurodiagnostico

Mision de Santo Tomas 1525-204
Zona del Rio
Tijuana, B.C. 22320
Mexico

011-5366-842-992

P.O. Box 431044
San Diego, California 92143-1044
United States

Contact Person

Salvador Rubio Veliz, M.D.

Background

Dr. Salvador Rubio Veliz is an M.D., specializing in neurology.

Illness Treated

Some cancers, Bell's palsy, herpes zoster, methadone addiction, epilepsy, and chronic gastric ulcers.

Treatment Offered

Chelation and combination of medicines and plants.

Length of Treatment/Stay

Three to six weeks.

Costs

Please call from 8 a.m. to 2 p.m. and 4 p.m. to 7 p.m. for information.

Method of Payment

The patient pays the center, and then collects from insurance.

Elisabeth-Anne Cole, M.D.

1002 Brockman
Sweeny, Texas 77480
United States

(409) 548-8610

Contact Person

Kathy Lane.

Primary Personnel

Elisabeth-Anne Cole, M.D., Ph.D., training in acupuncture, neural therapy, and sclerotherapy.

Directions

From Houston, Texas, take 288 South towards Angleton. Exit Highway 35 West Colombia (right turn). Continue through West Colombia on Highway 35 to C.R. 1459, and turn left. Continue on C.R. 1459 to Sweeny Hospital. Turn right on Alice Street, left on Ross Street, and right on Brockman. The clinic is the fifth house on the left.

Background

This clinic provides outpatient care, with treatments, lab work, interviews, etc., performed on the first visit. All treatments and therapies are specialized for each patient, with a holistic approach contributing to a high rate of improvement and remission.

Illness Treated

Immune dysfunction presenting as cancer—all phases, all tumors, at any location in the body. Also AIDS, HIV virus, lupus, multiple sclerosis, Parkinson's disease, rheumatoid arthritis, chronic fatigue syndrome, Crohn's disease, diabetes, atherosclerosis, hypertension, and fibromyalgia.

Treatment Offered

Nontoxic immune system enhancement and balancing to enable the body to seek out and destroy unhealthy cells and regenerate new cell reproduction through nutritional supplementation, diet, detoxification, oxygenation, and bioenergetic/electromagnetic strengthening. Therapy can begin at the first visit with optimum consecutive treatments continuing daily for fourteen to twenty-one days with a one-month follow-up program. Many modalities and supplemental combinations are used, designed for each individual patient daily. Pain control is also available.

Length of Treatment/Stay

Daily IV supplementation for fourteen to twenty-one days optimum treatment, with weekly follow-up for three months. Treatments and therapies vary daily and may be varied in length of time also, due to the individuality of the program. Recommended limited stay is two weeks. Maintenance program and instruction are implemented on the first visit.

Costs

Approximately $1,000 to $1,500 for the first week, including lab, office visit, IVs, and oral supplementation. Total for the optimum program is approximately $4,000.

Method of Payment

Cash, checks, traveler's checks, or cashier's checks are accepted. Insurance companies will reimburse for office visits and lab fees. Some companies will also reimburse for IV therapies. Medicare will reimburse for office visits and some lab fees.

Ernesto Contreras Jr., M.D.

2976 Paseo Playas Secc. Jardines del Sol, Playas
Playas de Tijuana, B.C. 22206
Mexico

011-526-680-9292
Fax: 011-526-680-9292

Mailing Address:
539 Telegraph Canyon Road
Suite 642
Chula Vista, California 91910
United States

Contact Person

Dr. Ernesto Contreras Jr., M.D.; Martha Salazar, secretary.

Primary Personnel

Dr. Contreras, oncologist; Francisco Espinosa, M.D., cancer surgeon; Jorge Astiazaran, M.D., internist; Gustavo Andrade, M.D., oncologist.

Directions

Take California Freeway 5 south to Tijuana, Mexico. Follow signs to Ensenada Toll Road, exit on Playas de Tijuana. Pass four lights and three more blocks. The facility is a six-story glass building on the left.

Background

After doing research at Hospital Ernesto Contreras for over thirty years, and treating more than 45,000 patients, in January 1996, it was decided to open a cancer research center for alternative cancer treatments, without the pressure from the busy hospital practice. More than forty-five M.D.s collaborate at this center under the direction of Dr. Ernesto Contreras Jr.

Illness Treated

Cancer.

Treatment Offered

Metabolic laetrile therapy, Warburg therapy, reduced dose conventional therapies, and immunotherapy. Alternative therapies are under research.

Length of Treatment/Stay

Three to six weeks.

Costs

$5,000 to $10,000, not including the cost of conventional therapies.

Method of Payment

Cash, money order, and checks with proper I.D. are accepted. Pre-approved insurance is accepted.

Cose Inc.
(Centre d'Orthobiologie Somatidienne de l'Estrie Inc.)

5270 Mills Street
Rock Forest, Quebec J1N 3B6
Canada

(819) 564-7883
Fax: (819) 564-4668
Internet: www.cose.com
E-mail: fguerin@cose.com

Primary Personnel

Gaston Naessens, Francoise Naessens, Stephane Sdicu, Daniel Sdicu, Andre Sdicu.

Directions

From Newport, Vermont, take Highway 55 after crossing the border, or Highway 10 East if coming from Montreal, always following indications for Sherbrooke. Take Exit 128 and turn right on Bertrand Fabi Street (third traffic light). Mills Street is two-and-a-half miles further on your right.

Background

More than forty years ago, Gaston Naessens invented the Somatoscope, a microscope capable of reaching 30,000X magnification with a 15nm resolution on living blood samples. Since then, Mr. Naessens has developed a condenser permitting ultramicroscopy. The condenser is adaptable to most microscopes, and available to all health care professionals. The Ultramicroscope makes it possible to observe processes in freshly extracted blood and to view its subcellular components. Gaston Naessens hypothesizes that all living beings, animal and vegetable, possess life by virtue of microscopic dense particles that he calls "somatids." His unique approach to studying morphological correlates of health from blood samples relies on using his Somatoscope and Ultramicroscope to view the abnormal cycle of the somatids in the blood (orthodox medicine has no live blood test for cancer). Studies in standardizing this blood test are presently in progress. Eventually, the results of these studies may lead to the elaboration of a blood test for diagnostic purposes and meet the approval requirements of the Canadian medical authorities. The center believes that cancer development is related to a lowering of inhibitors (e.g. chalones) transported in the blood.

Illness Treated

Cancer, multiple sclerosis, progressive rheumatoid arthritis, chronic fatigue syndrome, and other degenerative diseases.

Treatment Offered

714X (trimethylbicyclonitraminoheptane chloride). This medicine is a nitrogenated camphor-derivative mixed with mineral salts. The goal is to fluidify the lymph, and to direct nitrogen to the cancerous cells in order to stop their toxic secretions, which block the organism's defense mechanism. The use of 714X is authorized in Canada by the Health Protection Branch, Ottawa, in conformity with article C.08.010 of the Food and Drug Law (Emergency Drug Section). Any Canadian doctor can obtain 714X by requesting an authorization to use this product from the Health Protection Branch.

Related Readings

The Persecution and Trial of Gaston Naessens by Christopher Bird, 1991.

The Galileo of the Microscope by Christopher Bird, 1990.

AIDS, Cancer, and the Medical Establishment by Dr. Raymond Keith Brown, 1986.

The Somatidian Theory by Gaston Naessens, 1984. (A 45-minute VHS videocassette.)

Somatidian Orthobiology by Gaston Naessens, 1991. (A 55-minute VHS cassette.)

AIDS and the Somatidian Theory by Gaston Naessens, 1992. (A 27-minute VHS cassette.)

714X: Injection Technique by Gaston Naessens, 1994. (A 12-minute VHS cassette.)

Length of Treatment/Stay

714X is injected daily (perinodular). A series of shots consists of twenty-one daily injections; three such series are the minimum required, but most patients should expect to undergo longer-term treatment.

Costs

Enough medicine for one series of shots costs $320 in United States funds. Delivery takes only a few days. Included with the medicine are a protocol, injection instructions, and a videocassette on the treatment.

Method of Payment

Payment must be accompanied by a medical prescription. Checks and money orders made out to Cose Inc. are accepted. The medicine will not be mailed to post office boxes. Full name, address, and telephone number must accompany prescription and payment.

Cydel Medical Center

Bravlio Maldonado #1 Fracc. Soler
Tijuana, B.C. 22000
Mexico

(800) 248-8431

Mailing Address:
P.O. Box 434290
San Ysidro, California 92143
United States

(800) 433-4962

Contact Person

Mrs. Hilda Villasenor, or Mrs. Georgette Del Rio.

Primary Personnel

Jorge Vazquez, M.D.; Martha Sanchez, M.D.

Directions

Cross the border to Mexico, then take the Ensenada Road.

Background

The clinic has been in business for nineteen years.

Illness Treated

Cancer, multiple sclerosis, chronic fatigue syndrome, arthritis, Alzheimer's disease, and gout.

Treatment Offered

Laetrile, ozone therapy, colonics, massages, and others.

Related Readings

Death of Cancer by Harold Manner, Ph.D.

Length of Treatment/Stay

At least three weeks; fourth week is free.

Costs

The cost of stay varies depending on the treatment program and the addition of any services not included in the program. Once the patient has spoken to a doctor at the hospital and received a treatment recommendation, a hospital representative can estimate much of the cost for the patient.

Method of Payment

Cash, traveler's checks, cashier's checks, Visa, and MasterCard are accepted. The center works with Worldwide Insurance Coordinators, an insurance consulting firm that has experienced success in getting insurance companies to cover medical treatments received in Mexico. For all insurance questions, call Cydel Medical Center at (800) 433-4962.

Environmental and Preventive Health Center of Atlanta

3833 Roswell Road, Suite 110
Atlanta, Georgia 30342
United States

(404) 841-0088

Contact Person
Rachel Allen.

Primary Personnel
Stephen B. Edelson, M.D.

Directions
Buckhead, Atlanta. About five miles south of I-285 on Roswell Road.

Background
The center offers a choice of a comprehensive array of alternative adjunctive cancer therapies.

Illness Treated
All forms of cancer and other chronic diseases. The center also specializes in preventive aspects of cancer.

Treatment Offered
Preventive nutrition and various nontoxic treatments, including ultraviolet blood irradiation, intravenous hydrogen peroxide, vitamin C, amygdalin (laetrile), coffee enemas, shark cartilage, and others.

Length of Treatment/Stay
Varies; some patients spend six hours daily at the center, others receive only home therapy. The center obtains control of the cancer, then uses a maintenance program.

Costs
Varies from $800 to $12,000 monthly.

Method of Payment
Cash, check, Visa, and MasterCard are accepted No insurance is accepted directly, but the center will help patients file their claims.

Europa Institute of Integrated Medicine

Allen W. Lloyd Building, Suite 201
406 Avenue Paseo de Tijuana
International Border Zone
Tijuana, B.C.
Mexico

011-526-682-4902
Fax: 011-526-682-4920

United States Office:
P.O. Box 950
Twin Peaks, California 92391
United States

(909) 336-3671

Contact Person

Dr. Carolyn Bormann, United States office number; Dr. Jeffrey Freeman, Mexico number.

Primary Personnel

Jeffrey Freeman, M.D., founder; Sonia Rodriguez, M.D.; Carolyn Bormann, N.D.

Directions

Take I-5 or I-805 south to Mexican border. After coming out of border shute, take right fork, pull into first drive; Allen Lloyd Building is a six-story brown stucco.

Background

Dr. Freeman is an American physician who did his residency at Baylor. He and his wife, Dr. Rodriguez, have been involved in complementary/alternative medicine for over ten years, and believe in practicing according to the dictates of their consciences, not "cookbook" or "consensus" medicine; they also believe in keeping an open mind, and using a team approach with the patient. All viable, validated, scientifically-based approaches are used.

Illness Treated

All cancers; multiple sclerosis; lupus; CFIDS; viral syndromes; detoxification and rejuvenation program; allergies and immune dysfunctions.

Treatment Offered

Ozone, peroxide, chelation, photoluminescence, UBI, classical hyperthermia, amino acid and enzyme therapy, biologicals, homeopathy, naturopathy, functional and clinical nutrition, colon hydrotherapy, massage, bioelectric/polarity therapy, psycho-neuroimmunology, neural therapy, heavy metals and dental nerotoxin removals and detoxification.

Related Readings

Into the Light by William Campbell Douglass, M.D.

The Cancer Solution by Robert Wilner, M.D.

The Chelation Way by Morton Walker.

Root Canal Coverup by Dr. Menig.

It's All in Your Head by Hal Huggins.

Oxygen Therapy by Robert Altman and Ed McCabe.

Length of Treatment/Stay

Outpatient clinic only. Two to four weeks, six days per week (Monday to Saturday).

Costs

Average $300 to $500 per day.

Method of Payment

Cash and checks are accepted. Prepayment is necessary. The institute can work with an insurance administrator. The institute contracts to get reimbursed, and the administrator takes a 20 percent fee out of recovery funds.

Florida Preventive Health Services, Inc.

3902 Henderson Boulevard, Suite 206
Tampa, Florida 33629
United States

(813) 832-3220
Fax: (813) 573-4489

4908-A Creekside Drive
Clearwater, Florida 34620
United States

(813) 573-3775

Contact Person

Donald J. Carrow, M.D.; Richard DeFreitas, R.N.

Primary Personnel

Donald J. Carrow, M.D., medical director; Michael DeLorenzio, Ph.D., clinical nutritionist.

Directions

South on Dale Mabry Highway (exit) from I-275 in Tampa. At the corner of Dale Mabry and Henderson, turn south, one block to Church; clinic is on the corner of Henderson and Church.

Background

Founded in 1980 to serve the Tampa Bay area, the clinic provides an integrated approach to the treatment of cancer using nutritional and metabolic support infusions, dietary counseling, and immune stimulation, along with conventional methods, should the patient desire to use both approaches.

Illness Treated

Most forms of cancer.

Treatment Offered

Metabolic intravenous therapy, nutritional support, vaccine immune stimulation, Coley's mixed toxins, detoxification programs.

Related Readings

Cancer Therapy and Questioning Chemotherapy by Dr. Ralph Moss.
Cancer and Nutrition by John Boik.

Length of Treatment/Stay

Four weeks.

Costs

$50 to $200/infusion—all prices discussed in advance.

Method of Payment

Cash, check, Visa, MasterCard, and Discover are accepted. Insurance is accepted with written pre-authorization—insurance filed for all visits.

Foundation for Cartilage and Immunology Research

104 Post Office Road
Waccabuc, New York 10597
United States

(914) 763-6195
Fax: (914) 763-3342

Contact Person

Dr. John F. Prudden or Mrs. Jennifer DeFranco.

Primary Personnel

John F. Prudden, M.D., chairman and director; Mrs. Jennifer DeFranco, administrative assistant.

Directions

Call for directions.

Background

The foundation was established to perform basic biomedical laboratory work to identify the molecular entities responsible for the immunostimulatory, wound-healing acceleratory, and anti-inflammatory characteristics of bovine cartilage, when administered in appropriate dosage forms in clinical and laboratory settings. The consultants and directors of the foundation have expertise in basic research, and clinical investigation is conducted by Dr. Prudden.

Illness Treated

Bovine cartilage is used as a first-line therapy where other modalities are of little or no value, such as cancer of the pancreas, adenocarcinoma of the lung, squamous cell cancer of pharynx, lung, larynx (metastatic), renal cell carcinoma, and others. It is used as a reserve therapy in malignancies for which there are standard therapies of recognized effectiveness, such as breast, gastrointestinal, or prostate cancer.

Treatment Offered

At present, 9 gm/day is given (eight capsules containing 375 mg, with meals three times per day). Various methods have been devised for situations where this cannot be done.

Related Readings

Dr. Prudden has written several articles on the treatment of cancer with bovine cartilage.

Length of Treatment/Stay

Varies according to the patient.

Costs

Cost includes $200 initial consultation fee (a one-time charge for those advised by tele-phone; this group can call without charge thereafter). Visits to Dr. Prudden are $200 for initial visit, and $100 thereafter. Frequency of visits varies depending on circumstances. Cost of bovine cartilage is $187.50 per month.

Method of Payment

Checks are accepted. Patients pay initially, but every effort is made to help them collect on their insurance. The cost of the bovine cartilage is often paid if no standard treatment is available.

GenesisWest Research Institute for Biological Medicine

United States Agent:
P.O. Box 3460
Chula Vista, California 91909-0004
United States

(619) 424-9552
Fax: (619) 424-7593
Internet: www.cancertherapies.com

Clinic:
Avenida del Aqua 256
Secc. Jardines Fracc
Playas de Tijuana
Tijuana, B.C.
Mexico

Contact Person

Jacob Swilling, Ph.D., consultant.

Primary Personnel

Sergio Amescua, M.D., and four other physicians, supported by a staff of nurses.

Directions

GenesisWest offers a courtesy driver service to meet patients at the San Diego Airport. Reception: Calle Roca #1340 Secc., Jardines, Fracc., Playas de Tijuana, Tijuana, Baja California, Mexico. Telephone: 011-5266-301313. If you are driving: once you cross the border, you will see on your right-hand side several places to buy insurance; you *must* have insurance to drive in Mexico. Follow the sign to "Ensenada/Rosarito." Watch for a sign reading "Playas" on your right, then pass the bullring on the right. You pass the El Cortez Motel and a vacant lot on the right. Turn right at the stop light into Avenida del Aqua. Make another right at the next corner; the entrance is here.

Background

GenesisWest was established six years ago as a research and healing center based on the work of scientist Jacob Swilling, Ph.D., internationally known for his work in biological medicine. The major focus of this clinic is its emphasis on the need to reveal the origin of the disease, typically multicausal. Advanced technology is used to reveal imbalances in all systems, then to determine the source of these imbalances. Treatment is customized to correct imbalances by correcting the source. The clinic operates on the philosophy that it is the body which heals itself. To maximize healing, body balance needs to be restored. The clinic offers intensive inpatient care as well as a three-day predictive medicine early warning detection program.

Illness Treated

Cancer and other degenerative diseases.

Treatment Offered

Intensive multifaceted treatment, combining ozone; ultraviolet blood irradiation; Rife frequency; hyperthermia; immunotherapy; IVs; amino acid/electrolyte and HCL pH balancing; DMSO; homeopathic, herbal, and botanical combinations; bioenergetic, eletromagnetic, and neural therapy; 714X; laetrile; enzyme and metabolic therapies; Eco colon restoration; B_{15}; and Germanium nebulizers.

Related Readings

pH and Electrolyte Balance as a Health-Determining Factor by Jacob Swilling, Ph.D.

Mounting Evidence Charts the Direction for Future Development in Biological Medicine Used in Treatment of Cancer and Other Diseases by Jacob Swilling, Ph.D.

Audio tapes: *Predictive Medicine; Early Warning Detection to Avoid a Later Crisis;* and *New Dimensions in Cancer Control.*

Length of Treatment/Stay

Minimum three weeks for cancer and degenerative diseases. One-, three-, and six-day predictive medicine programs.

Costs

Range from $980 for one-day predictive medicine evaluation to $3,800 per week. Treatment programs include spouse or companion sharing private suite with two beds, and meals.

Method of Payment

Traveler's checks, cash, and bank transfer are accepted. Payments must be made each week for weekly programs. To determine whether you are eligible for insurance refund, call IHCR for information: (619) 575-7684.

Gerson Healing Centers of America

Gerson Center at Sedona
Sedona, Arizona
United States

Gerson Institute (call for information and admissions):
P.O. Box 430
Bonita, California 91902
United States

(619) 585-7600
Fax: (619) 585-7610
Internet: www.gerson.org
E-mail: info@gerson. org

Contact Person

Ask for the Client Services Department.

Primary Personnel

Homeopathic medical doctors and registered nurses, offering twenty-four-hour skilled care.

Directions

Call the Gerson Institute.

Background

The center offers nutritional healing based on the Gerson therapy. Together, the doctors have over thirty years' experience with this therapy, with excellent results. Lectures and demonstrations are given in Gerson therapy techniques, food and juice preparation, and other topics.

Illness Treated

Primarily all forms of cancer, but also all chronic, degenerative diseases, especially heart disease, diabetes, multiple sclerosis, lupus, high blood pressure, rheumatoid arthritis, chronic fatigue, liver diseases, colitis, Crohn's disease, and others.

Treatment Offered

The full Gerson therapy is offered, including thirteen glasses of freshly prepared juices. All foods are from organic fruits and vegetables. Intensive detoxification is given, including coffee enemas. Minerals, enzymes, liver extract, B_{12}, and other supplements are offered. Adjunctive therapies are available, including acupuncture, chiropractic, massage, botanicals, and others.

Related Readings

Healing Cancer and Other Degenerative Diseases With the Gerson Therapy by Charlotte Gerson and Chip White. Gerson Institute, 1997.

Cancer Winner by Jacquie Davison. Gerson Institute, 1989.

A Time to Heal by Beata Bishop. Penguin Worldwide, 1996.

Length of Treatment/Stay

The average stay is three weeks, but depending on the severity of the illness, patients may stay from two to six weeks. At-home therapy lasts for one to two years, depending on the condition.

Costs

All-inclusive cost is $4,895 per week for the patient and a companion. For the patient, this includes: private room and bath; all thirteen juices and meals; all medical visits, treatments, medication, and nursing; teas; coffee for enemas; lectures; free books and videotapes; massages, acupuncture, and other adjunctive therapies; fresh fruit plate in room daily; and all organic materials. Blood tests and urinalysis are also included. Companion receives twin bed in the patient's, room and three vegetarian Gerson meals, including a glass of juice at each meal.

Method of Payment

Credit cards, cash, or traveler's checks are accepted. Insurance assignments cannot be accepted. Insurance processing is available.

Gerson Institute
(Hospital Meridien de Playas de Tijuana)

Calle de Lava 2971
Secc. Costa Hermosa
Playas de Tijuana, B.C.
Mexico

Gerson Institute (call for information and admissions):
P.O. Box 430
Bonita, California 91902
United States

(619) 585-7600
Fax: (619) 585-7610
Internet: www.gerson.org
E-mail: info@gerson.org

Contact Person

Ask for the Client Services Department.

Primary Personnel

Five to six fully licensed medical doctors, at least one on duty twenty-four hours, as well as registered nurses.

Directions

Call the Gerson Institute.

Background

The hospital offers nutritional healing based on the Gerson therapy. Together, the doctors have over thirty years' experience with this therapy, with excellent results. Lectures and demonstrations are given almost daily in Gerson therapy techniques, food and juice preparation, and other topics.

Illness Treated

All chronic, degenerative diseases; mainly all forms of cancer. Excellent responses are also seen in high blood pressure, heart disease, diabetes, chronic fatigue, liver diseases, lupus, rheumatoid arthritis, colitis, Crohn's diseases, multiple sclerosis, and others.

Treatment Offered

The full Gerson therapy is offered, including thirteen glasses of freshly prepared juices. All foods are from organic fruits and vegetables. Intensive detoxification is given, including coffee enemas. Minerals, enzymes, liver extract, B_{12}, pancreatic enzymes, and other supplements are offered. Adjunctive therapies include hyperthermia, acupuncture, massage, laetrile, and botanicals.

Related Readings

Cancer Winner by Jacquie Davison. Gerson Institute, 1989.

Healing Cancer and Other Degenerative Diseases With the Gerson Therapy by Charlotte Gerson and Chip White. Gerson Institute, 1997.

A Time to Heal by Beata Bishop. Penguin Worldwide, 1996.

Length of Treatment/Stay

Most cancer patients' suggested stay is three weeks; other patients occasionally can be accepted for two weeks; extremely ill persons extend their stay from four to six weeks. At-home therapy needs to be carried on for one to two years, depending on condition.

Costs

All-inclusive cost is $4,500 per week. This includes: private room and bath, all thirteen juices and meals, all medical visits and treatments, all medication and nursing, teas, coffee for enemas, lectures, free books and videotapes, massages, hyperthermia, acupuncture, fresh fruit plate in room daily, and all organic materials.

Method of Payment

For the first two weeks, cash or traveler's checks are accepted. At the beginning of the third week, credit card payments can be accepted. Insurance assignments cannot be accepted. Insurance processing is available.

Gerson Research Organization
(In collaboration with the Max Gerson Memorial Cancer Center of Centro Hospitalario Internacional Pacifico, S.A. de C.V.)

Gerson Research Organization:
7807 Artesian Road
San Diego, California 92127-2117
United States

(800) 759-2966 (U.S.A.)
(800) 754-0466 (Canada)
04-737-761620 (U.K.)

Centro Hospitalario Internacional Pacifico, S.A. de C.V. (CHIPSA):
Max Gerson Memorial Cancer Center
670 Nubes
Playas de Tijuana, B.C.
Mexico

Contact Person

Gar Hildenbrand, president.

Primary Personnel

Dan E. Rogers, M.D., co-principal investigator and chief of the cancer center; Gar Hildenbrand, co-principal investigator and chief of clinical epidemiology; Josef Issels, M.D., co-principal investigator and consulting physician; Ron Carreño, M.D., chief of hyperbaric medicine; Rafael Cedeño, M.D., medical director; Christeene Hildenbrand, project director.

Directions

The hospital provides transportation from San Diego's airport, train and bus stations, hotels, and motels. From the U.S. Highway 5 and 805 border crossing in San Ysidro, California, follow the clearly posted signs west toward Ensenada. At the crest of a steep hill, the road turns left and descends into a valley. As you reach the floor of the valley, turn right at the Playas exit. Follow this road through a pass in the foothills. As the ocean becomes visible, look for the first stoplight, which marks Paseo Ensenada. Turn left here and proceed approximately 1.2 miles (ten long blocks) to Nubes; turn right. CHIPSA is one block to the right.

Background

The Gerson Research Organization was formed in 1993 to provide a clinical epidemiological component to the long-standing collaboration of CHIPSA and its former partner, the Gerson Institute. Research findings led to dramatic changes in CHIPSA's medical practice, and to conflicts in treatment philosophy, which were resolved with the departure of the Gerson Institute in early 1996. After eighteen years, 7,000 charts of patients treated with Gerson's diet therapy have been collected. Analyses led to the general conclusion that this therapy should be put into a larger, multidisciplinary context. The first planned experimental effort involved integration of Gerson's therapy with Dr. Evangelos Danopoulos' urea/creatine protocols for cancer. The preclinical impressions recorded were so far beyond expectation, including regressions of tumors chronically resistant to diet therapy alone, that CHIPSA/GRO began to search for additional well-documented and promising treatments. The mixed bacterial vaccine of Dr. William B. Coley was introduced next, and again the preliminary data were very gratifying. Dr. Josef Issels joined the CHIPSA/GRO collaboration in mid-1996 as a co-principal investigator, and permission was quickly obtained from the Mexican government to offer Dr. Issels' autogenous specific cancer vaccines. At the same time, negotiations were completed with representatives of Russian immunologist Constantin Govallo, M.D., developer of immunoembryological therapy (placental extract vaccines). All treatments are integrated, according to prior experience with and outcomes of the Gerson therapy, and by the Issels "Pathogenesis of Cancer Hypothesis," which provides a template for integration of multiple disciplines in the management of advanced cancer.

Illness Treated

The primary research focus has been cancer. However, many of the treatments used are pro-host in nature. Experience has taught that many degenerative diseases, including autoimmunities, CHD, Type II diabetes, and some central nervous system diseases will also respond to multidisciplinary management. Medical guidance has been frequently requested by individuals seeking to turn back the syndromes associated with aging, including weight gain, fatigue, mental deterioration, and failing physical functions.

Treatment Offered

The program for cancer has three major components:

1. Pro-host therapies. These are centered around Gerson's diet therapy and Issels' treatments and include UV blood irradiation, homeopathic medicines, patient-specific supplemental micronutrients, botanicals, ozone, hyperbaric oxygen, and hyperthermia.

2. Anti-tumor treatments. Although Gerson's therapy with additional supportive treatments has been observed to cause regression of disease, often patients need far more treatment, including any reasonable effort to shrink or remove tumors. Danopoulos' protocols with urea and creatine are used extensively as a nontoxic method of regressing tumors. In some cases, surgery may be advisable to lower tumor bulk. Chemotherapy and radiation are at the bottom of the hierarchy of resorts, but can be used judiciously if needed. They are never given chronically, but are instead treated as short-term alternatives or complements to surgery. They are followed by intensive pro-host treatment and immunotherapy. Surgery, chemotherapy, and radiation are not regarded as potentially curative treatments, and have been put in a much broader context in CHIPSA.

3. Immunotherapy. Aggressive immunotherapy treatments will include the famous "toxins" of Coley, as well as autogenous mycoplasma vaccines prepared under the direction of Dr. Issels. Govallo's VG1000 placental extract vaccines are being studied in a special prospective evaluation.

Related Readings

Hildenbrand GLG, Hildenbrand C, Bradford K, Rogers D, Straus C, Cavin S. "The role of follow-up and retrospective data analysis in alternative cancer management: the Gerson experience." *Journal of Naturopathic Medicine* 1996: in press.

Hildenbrand GLG, Hildenbrand. "Defining the role of diet therapy in complementary cancer management: prevention of recurrence vs. regression of disease." *Proceedings of the First Annual Alternative Therapies Symposium: Creating Integrated Healthcare.* January 18-20, 1996, San Diego, CA.

Hildenbrand GLG, Hildenbrand C, Bradford K, Cavin S. "Five-year survival rates of melanoma patients treated by diet therapy after the manner of Gerson." *Alt. Ther. Health. Med.* 1995; I(4): 29-37.

Hildenbrand GLG, Chair, contributing author, editorial review board. "Diet and Nutrition in the Prevention and Treatment of Chronic Disease (chapter)." *Alternative Medicine: Expanding Medical Horizons.* NIH Publication No. 94-066; U.S. Government Printing Office, December, 1994.

Hildenbrand GLG, Lechner P. "A reply to Saul Green's critique of the rationale for cancer treatment with coffee enemas and diet: cafestol derived from beverage coffee increases bile production in rats; and coffee enemas and diet ameliorate human cancer pain in stages I and II." *Townsend Letter for Doctors.* May, 1994.

Hess DJ. *Can Bacteria Cause Cancer? Politics and the Evaluation of Alternative Medicine.* New York; New York University Press: 1997.

Hildenbrand GLG, *Key Concepts in Science Studies.* New York; New York University Press: 1997.

Length of Program/Stay

Varies according to the case and to individual resources. Five to six weeks are recommended based on the need to prepare patients for immunotherapy. Because hospitalization is more expensive than outpatient care, and because a primary care physician near the patient's home can be so helpful, CHIPSA will cooperate with, and provide practical information to, home-based practitioners (M.D.s, D.O.s, N.D.s, D.C.s, etc.). When a local primary care physician can initiate Gerson's non-proprietary therapy along with other appropriate supportive measures to prepare the patient for immunotherapy, patients can shorten their CHIPSA stay by several weeks. In the case of naturopaths who are not allowed to administer certain prescription drugs, an earlier version of Gerson's therapy with modern supplementation can be used. On referral to CHIPSA, its physicians will prescribe the case-appropriate controlled materials, including immunotherapy vaccines, as tertiary care specialists. CHIPSA will then refer the patient home to the primary care physician.

Costs

A deposit of $3,000 (U.S.) plus 10 percent sales and service tax for the patient, and $308 plus 10 percent tax for a companion, are required for admission. This is not a flat fee; costs will be affected by the number and type of complementary treatments required or desired by the physician and/or the patient. Based on stage and complications of each patient, costs for five weeks may range from $20,000 upward. Costs can be lowered if regional primary care practitioners join in a cooperative effort as described above.

Method of Payment

Costs of conventional procedures, such as surgery, diagnostics, and hospitalization, are normally reimbursable by private insurance. CHIPSA does not file insurance forms, and no insurance assignments have been made. Therefore, reimubursement must be sought by the individual. Several firms offer assistance seeking reimbursement.

Nicholas Gonzalez, M.D.

36A East 36th Street
New York, New York 10016
United States

(212) 213-3337
Fax: (212) 213-3414

Primary Personnel

Nicholas J. Gonzalez, M.D.; Linda L. Isaacs, M.D.

Directions

The office is located between Park and Madison Avenues in midtown Manhattan. Please do not go to the office without an appointment; prospective patients should feel free to call for more information.

Background

Dr. Gonzalez and Dr. Isaacs provide an intensive nutritional program, which involves diet, nutritional supplementation, and detoxification. Each protocol is highly individualized. The initial evaluation requires two sessions; out-of-town patients must come to New York to be evaluated. The first meeting involves a complete history and physical examination, and usually takes an hour. The second session takes approximately an hour and a half; during this session, the doctor reviews in depth his evaluation and the results of various tests. In addition, he reviews the patient's diet, supplement, and detoxification programs. Before an appointment can be made, prospective patients must relay the details of their case to the office in a ten- to fifteen-minute interview with our staff. Dr. Gonzalez and Dr. Isaacs then review this material, to be sure that the patient's diagnosis, current condition, and extent of previous treatment will not prevent him or her from benefiting from this approach. It is necessary for the patients themselves to call; not only does this give the staff more accurate information, but it also helps insure that the patient understands the high degree of motivation and commitment the program demands. Patients who are currently receiving chemotherapy and/or radiation, are advised against following this program, as it has been found that patients who combine more than one approach do not get the full benefit of any of the programs.

Illness Treated

Dr. Gonzalez and Dr. Isaacs treat a wide variety of disorders, but their primary research interest is cancer. They currently do not treat HIV-related disorders.

Treatment Offered

This program involves individualized diet, supplementation, and detoxification. Diets vary widely, from vegetarian diets to those high in animal protein, but all diets require the use of unprocessed, organically grown foods. In addition, patients will be required to give up the use of alcohol and tobacco. The supplements consist of vitamins, minerals, enzymes, and glandular concentrates; a cancer patient may take as many as 150 capsules per day. In addition to the diet and supplements, each program involves a variety of detoxification procedures. These are techniques, such as coffee enemas, that help clear the body of metabolic wastes. We find that these procedures are critically important to the success of the nutritional program.

Related Readings

The program and its theory are described more thoroughly in a tape recording of a lecture given by Dr. Gonzalez. This can be obtained by calling Willner's Pharmacy in New York at (212) 685-0448 or (800) 633-1106, Monday through Friday between 9 a.m. and 7 p.m., and on Saturday between 9 a.m. and 5 p.m. Another tape regarding this therapy is available from the World Research Foundation at (818) 907-5483.

Length of Treatment/Stay

The patient is instructed on what to do during the initial visits, then follows the various procedures at home. The total duration of the program varies from patient to patient. Patients are encouraged to view this program as a long-term lifestyle change.

Costs

The total charge for the initial sessions is $1,800. This also covers the time taken to design the protocol. The fee does not include the costs of any required blood tests. We do not charge for phone service; we expect patients to feel free to call as needed. We have worked the cost of phone consultations into the initial fee. The supplements are not sold in the office, but are available through mail order. The charge varies from patient to patient, but will run about $400 per month for a cancer patient. All together, a cancer patient will spend about $6,000 per year to follow this treatment.

Method of Payment

Cash, personal checks (U.S. funds on U.S. bank), or traveler's checks are accepted. Patients are responsible for paying their bills at the time of service. Insurance coverage varies, but due to the nature of the work, many companies, including Medicare and Medicaid, will not reimburse for any part of the services.

Dayton Haigney, M.D.

46 Dow Highway
Eliot, Maine 03903
United States

(207) 439-1068

Contact Person

Dayton F. Haigney, M.D.

Primary Personnel

Dayton F. Haigney, M.D.

Directions

46 Route 236, Eliot, Maine. Across the street from the Eliot Commons Shopping Center. Rear entry.

Background

Dr. Haigney is a board certified specialist in physical medicine and rehabilitation. He integrates different conventional and alternative medicines in the management of chronic diseases.

Illness Treated

Chronic degenerative diseases, breast cancer, chronic fatigue syndrome, and fibromyalgia.

Treatment Offered

Homeopathy, osteopathic manipulation, acupuncture, hypnosis, nutrition, counseling, hydrogen peroxide, and herbal medicine.

Length of Treatment/Stay

Patients are evaluated for one-and-a-half hours initially, then seen for half-hour follow-ups as needed.

Costs

Initial consult: $150. Follow-up: $65. Acupuncture: $90.

Method of Payment

Cash, checks, Visa, and MasterCard are accepted.

Ross A. Hauser, M.D., D.C.

715 Lake, #600
Oak Park, Illinois 60301
United States

(708) 848-7789
Fax: (708) 848-7763

Primary Personnel

Marion A. Hauser, M.S., R.D., C.N.S.D., clinical dietician.

Illness Treated

Chronic pain, allergies, blockages of arteries, cancer, and chronic fatigue.

Treatment Offered

Bio-oxidative therapy (ozone, hydrogen peroxide), ream's testing, allergy testing, prolotherapy (an injection technique which helps reduce pain in cancer and arthritis patients), and photoluminescence (in which a certain amount of blood is drawn, exposed to ultraviolet light, and returned to the body).

Length of Treatment/Stay

Varies depending on the case. Prolotherapy is usually performed every six weeks, more often in acute cases.

Costs

Bio-oxidative therapy: $125 per treatment. IV hydrogen peroxide: $75 per treatment. Photoluminescence: $125 per treatment.

Method of Payment

Cash, checks, and credit cards are accepted. Insurance will usually cover initial consultation, office visits, and lab work, but other treatments may not be covered.

Health Achievement Center

112 S. 4th Street
Darby, Pennsylvania 19023-2809
United States

(610) 461-6225
Fax: (610) 558-5895

Pennsylvania Hospital Institute:
111 North 49th Street
Philadelphia, Pennsylvania 19139
United States

(215) 471-2000

Contact Person

Lance S. Wright, M.D.; Barbara Ramsay, R.N.; Faith Charles, Ph.D.

Primary Personnel

Barbara Ramsay, chelation and massage; Faith Charles, group and family counseling.

Directions

From 95 North, past Philadelphia, to Exit 12. Bartram to Island Avenue. Right turn, two miles to Bluebell Avenue. Turn left onto Main Street in Darby, to 4th Street. Turn left, go one-and-a-half blocks to 112 South 4th. From 95 South, exit 291 just before airport and go four miles. Left turn on Island Avenue, then two miles to Bluebell Avenue, then proceed as above.

Background

Dr. Wright, a founding member of the American Holistic Medical Association and certified in neuropsychiatry, established the center to treat the whole person with the latest comprehensive diagnostics. This is followed by indicated treatment to restore the balance of body chemistry and mental, psychological, and spiritual integrity. Patients also learn a healthy lifestyle to enhance immunity and sustain wellness.

Illness Treated

Degenerative diseases, including cancer, atherosclerosis, arthritis, toxic states, chronic fatigue, attention deficit disorder, substance abuse, depression, anxiety, mental illness, and psychosomatic problems.

Treatment Offered

Assessment of biological terrain, electroacupuncture, neural therapy, chelation, bio-oxidative therapy, hydrotherapy, psychotherapy, detoxification, and others.

Related Readings

Relaxation Response by Herbert Benson, M.D.

Reversing Heart Disease by Dean Ornish.

Perfect Health by Deepak Chopra, M.D.

Spontaneous Healing by Andrew Weil, M.D.

Journal of the American Preventive Medicine Association.

Journal of the American College for Advancement of Medicine.

Length of Treatment/Stay

Chelation, three hours. Bio-oxidation, one-and-a-half hours. Electroacupuncture, forty-five minutes. EMDR, one hour. Psychotherapy, one hour. Group therapy, one-and-a-half hours.

Costs

$60 to $150 for individual therapies. Full program varies from $300 to $2,500.

Method of Payment

Cash, checks, and Visa are accepted. The center is a provider for Blue Cross, Blue Shield, Prudential, Aetna, and GreenSpring on an individual basis.

Health Quest Clinic

24 High Street
Hampton, New Hampshire 03842
United States

(603) 929-4161

157 State Road
Kittery, Maine
United States

(207) 438-9372

Contact Person

Dr. Floyd W. S-R. Hoyt, N.D., D.Sc.

Directions

In Maine: I-95 to Exit 2, then south one block from Kittery Circle. In New Hampshire: I-95 to Hampton exit, then Route 101 east to Route 27 east, to Route 24. One mile to High Street.

Background

Health Quest is a center for natural medicine, dedicated to patients' maintenance of, and restoration to, optimum youthful health and vitality. The center integrates all the ancient forms with modern medicine and minor (cosmetic) surgery.

Illness Treated

Cancer, allergies, arthritis, asthma, back pain, chronic fatigue, headaches, hyperactivity, premenstrual syndrome, and others.

Treatment Offered

Homeopathy, all naturopathic modalities, nutrition, Chinese medicine, Ayurvedic medicine, acupressure, massage, and oxygen treatment.

Related Readings

Options by Walters.

Length of Treatment/Stay

Twelve weeks and up.

Costs

Costs are scheduled individually, but range from $2,000 and up for extensive cancer therapies over many weeks.

Method of Payment

Cash, checks, Visa, and MasterCard are accepted. The clinic will assist patients with insurance reimbursement.

The Hoffman Center

40 East 30th Street
10th Floor
New York, New York 10016
United States

(212) 779-1744

Contact Person

JoAnne Castagna or Helen Burgess.

Primary Personnel

Ronald L. Hoffman, M.D., medical director; Dr. Ilana Goldman, associate; Dr. Henry Hom, associate.

Directions

Located in midtown Manhattan, between Park Avenue and Madison Avenue.

Background

Dr. Hoffman: B.A. Columbia College, M.D. Einstein College. Dr. Goldman: B.A. Harvard, M.D. New York Medical College. Dr. Hom: M.D. SUNY Downstate Medical College.

Illness Treated

Cancer; also muscular degeneration, Lyme disease, irritable bowel syndrome, chronic fatigue syndrome, heart conditions, HIV, and asthma.

Treatment Offered

Complementary treatments for cancer. The center works alongside cancer specialists, providing nutritional support, and megadoses of vitamins in the form of intravenous infusions. Also available are chelation therapy, acupuncture, traditional Chinese medicine, extensive allergy treatment facilities, bee venom therapy for multiple sclerosis and arthritis, neural therapy for chronic pain, and nutritional counseling.

Length of Treatment/Stay

Varies.

Costs

Fees vary, depending on treatment.

Method of Payment

Cash, personal checks, and all major credit cards are accepted. Most insurance is accepted.

Holistic Medical Center

8264 Santa Monica Boulevard
Los Angeles, California 90046
United States

(213) 650-1789

537 East Ojai Avenue
Ojai, California 93023
United States

(805) 640-8080

Contact Person

Maria Levin.

Primary Personnel

Emil Levin, M.D., medical director.

Directions

On Santa Monica Boulevard between Fairfax and La Cienega.

Background

The center was established in Los Angeles in 1981. It uses European methods for cleansing and detoxifying the body, and minerals and vitamins to build the immune system.

Illness Treated

Viral diseases, parasites, allergies, asthma, digestive disorders, hepatitis, heart disease, premenstrual syndrome, diabetes, eczema, and dermatitis.

Treatment Offered

Colon therapy, infusion therapy, homeopathic treatments, viral and parasite treatments, chelation therapy, desensitization with homeopathic method for environmental and food allergies, mineral balancing, vitamin injections, neural therapy, and spider vein treatments.

Length of Treatment/Stay

Individually tailored to each patient.

Costs

Initial visit: $125 for approximately one hour. Regular visits: $85. Infusion therapy: $85 to $105. Chelation therapy: $85. Colonics: $65 to $75.

Method of Payment

Cash and checks are accepted. Insurance from several companies is accepted.

Hospital Bajanor S.A. de C.V.

Calle Ferrocarril, #10634
Tijuana, B.C.
Mexico

011-5266-823-005
Fax: 011-5266-823-006
Mailing Address:
P.O. Box 430531
San Diego, California 92143

(618) 975-3166
E-mail: carlosg@bbs.cincol.net

Contact Person

Dr. Carlos Alessandrini.

Directions

Patients should call for directions, or the clinic will pick them up at the border.

Background

The hospital was founded in 1990, and has been serving the community of Tijuana as a small, but full-service, emergency and outpatient hospital. Recently, the general director of Bajanor Hospital decided that his facility could better serve its purpose if its services were extended to provide a clinic that would rejuvenate and rebuild patients. By using the best of alternative medical technologies, the hospital endeavors to restore exhausted glandular and immune systems, and repair and rejuvenate patients to total, glowing health.

Illness Treated

Cancer, arthritis, heart disease, lung infections, urinary tract infections, kidney stones, and other degenerative diseases.

Treatment Offered

The treatment consists of first detoxifying the body so that energy is not wasted attempting to handle environmental poisons and other toxic materials. Then, emphasis is placed on rejuvenation using the best modalities. These include: polypeptides, EDTA chelation, amino acids, haematoxylon, laetrile, germanium, Hoxsey therapy, GH3, SV, DMSO peroxide, VIT drips, Sulconar and other live cell treatments, and nutrition and detoxification.

Length of Treatment/Stay

A basic treatment cycle consists of three weeks of outpatient treatment followed by an extensive re-evaluation of the patient's condition, to determine the extent of any further treatment, if needed.

Costs

Basic service is $275 per day, excluding certain diagnostic procedures and some special live cell therapies, if needed.

Method of Payment

Cash and checks are accepted. Insurance is accepted.

Hospital Santa Monica

Corporate Offices:
880 Canarios Court
Suite 210
Chula Vista, California 91910
United States

(800) 359-6547
(619) 428-1146

Hospital:
Avenida Mazatlan O/N
Rosarito Beach, B.C.
Mexico

011-526-613-3333

Contact Person

Hospital Santa Monica corporate offices are located in Chula Vista, California; the hospital itself is in Mexico. For reservations and information, call the office staff at (800) 359-6547.

Primary Personnel

Kurt W. Donsbach, D.C., N.D., Ph.D., founder and director; Humberto Seimandi, M.D., medical director; Richard Marsh, M.D.

Directions

Call for directions.

Background

Hospital Santa Monica was founded by Kurt W. Donsbach in 1987. Treatment is based on the premise that cancer and other chronic and degenerative diseases could be successfully treated using alternative methods, concentrating on bio-oxidative therapy, ultraviolet blood purification, hyperthermia, and a sugar-restricted diet.

Illness Treated

Cancer is the primary illness treated. Other chronic and degenerative diseases, such as candida, chronic fatigue syndrome, multiple sclerosis, heart disease, arthritis, and emphysema, are also treated.

Treatment Offered

Ozone and hydrogen peroxide, photoluminescence, nutritional therapy, bovine cartilage, hyperthermia, biomagnetics, colonics, IV chelation, and modified citrus pectin.

Related Readings

Wholistic Cancer Therapy by Kurt W. Donsbach, D.C., N.D., Ph.D.
Oxygen, Oxygen, Oxygen by Kurt W. Donsbach, D.C., N.D., Ph.D.
Oxygen Therapies by Ed McCabe.
Oxygen Healing Therapies by Nathaniel Altman.

Length of Treatment/Stay

For cancer and other chronic and degenerative diseases, twenty-one days. For detoxification, ten days. There are no outpatient therapies.

Costs

For cancer, $14,900. For other diseases (except multiple sclerosis), $8,400. For multiple sclerosis, $9,900. For detoxification, $2,900.

Method of Payment

Some insurance companies will cover at least part of the treatment. The hospital will bill insurance companies, with the exception of Medicare, Medicaid, HMOs, and Medicare supplements.

Richard P. Huemer, M.D.

3303 N.E. 44th Street
Vancouver, Washington 98663
United States

(800) 444-1696

c/o Hull Eye Center
1739 West Avenue J
Lancaster, California 93534
United States

(205) 253-4445
(503) 256-9666

Primary Personnel

Richard P. Huemer, M.D.

Directions

From Portland, Oregon: Go north on I-5 to State Route 500 (two miles beyond the river), then go east to the first light (St. John's). Turn left, go to the next light (which is 44th) and turn left again. The clinic is at the end of the block.

Background

Dr. Huemer has been involved full-time with nutritional and metabolic therapies since 1974. Previously, he was involved for nine years in research on cancer immunology. The clinic is an outpatient facility.

Illness Treated

Cancer, most degenerative diseases, atherosclerosis, chemical sensitivities, chronic fatigue syndrome, and autism.

Treatment Offered

Dr. Huemer does not treat cancer per se, but he provides nutritional support programs for cancer patients under the care of an oncologist. The support includes intravenous vitamin C, high-dose nutrient therapy, and immune stimulation. BCG is used as an adjunctive therapy in selected cases. Possible side effects are local scarring due to the BCG, and toxicity from vitamin A and selenium. Contact the office for specific instructions on how to prepare for an appointment and the tests that will be part of your first visit.

Related Readings

I Beat Cancer by Bernice Wallin. Contemporary Books, 1978.

Roots of Molecular Medicine by R.P. Huemer (editor). W.H. Freeman, 1986.

"The Healthy Heart Chart" by R.P. Huemer, M. McCarty, and H. Boynton. *Nutrition* 21, 1985.

Length of Treatment/Stay

Depends upon the situation.

Costs

Charges are based upon the amount of time spent. The initial visit costs about $100 (includes 30 percent discount for cash payment), plus office tests. Lab tests are extra and will be billed by the labs. Follow-up visits cost about $50. IVs range in price from $75 to $115.

Method of Payment

Cash, MasterCard, Visa, and Discover are accepted. The office does not presently bill insurance carriers. Patients are fully responsible for charges not covered by insurance. Payment at the time of service is requested.

Immuno-Augmentative Therapy Centre

P.O. Box F-42689
Freeport, Grand Bahama Island
Bahamas

(809) 352-7455
Fax: (809) 352-3201

P.O. Box 22579
Fort Lauderdale, Florida 33335
United States

Contact Person

John Clement, M.D.; June Austin; Edward Granger, administrator.

Primary Personnel

John Clement, M.D.; Lynn Austin, R.N.

Directions

In the center of Freeport, next to the Rand Hospital.

Background

The Immuno-Augmentative Therapy Centre was founded in 1977 by Dr. Lawrence Burton to treat various forms of cancer using naturally occurring proteins found in human blood serum. To date, more than 3,500 patients have sought control of their cancers using this form of treatment at the IAT Centre. In June 1996, the clinic expanded its treatments by contracting with Empirical Therapies, Inc., of Washington, D.C., to introduce VG-1000, a medicine made from human placenta, which was discovered by a Russian medical researcher and immunologist. Today, patients have a choice of either of these two therapies, depending on the type of cancer and its characteristics.

Illness Treated

All kinds of carcinomas, melanomas, mesotheliomas, lymphomas, Hodgkin's disease, sarcomas, and chronic lymphatic leukemia.

Treatment Offered

The immuno-augmentative therapy uses fractions of whole blood. The blood is taken daily from healthy volunteers (usually the family members of patients), and centrifuged to provide the elements needed for treatment. Very small amounts are injected daily for the duration of the treatment. Patients may expect to remain at the clinic for four to eight weeks at their first visit, and must return periodically for additional diagnosis and treatment. VG-1000 is made at the clinic from fresh placentas obtained after normal live births at local hospitals in Freeport (placentas from abortions are never used). It is administered in the form of two injections one week apart. The patient may return in two to three months for a booster shot if that appears necessary.

Related Readings

The clinic will provide materials on immuno-augmentative therapy. A good discussion of VG-1000 as a cancer therapy can be found in *Immunology of Pregnancy and Cancer* by Valentin I. Govallo. Commack, NY: Nova Science Publishers, 1993.

Length of Treatment/Stay

The patient receiving immuno-augmentative therapy must plan to remain in Freeport (as an outpatient) for eight to twelve weeks, and must return for a two-week monitoring period every four to six months thereafter. The patient receiving VG-1000 should plan to remain in Freeport for eight to ten days for the first visit, and there may be a requirement for a booster shot in two to three months.

Costs

The cost of immuno-augmentative therapy is $7,500 for the first four weeks, and $700 a week thereafter, for up to eight weeks. VG-1000 costs $8,500 for the first visit and $1,500 for a booster shot. Neither of these charges covers transportation to the Bahamas and room and board while in Freeport.

Method of Payment

Visa, MasterCard, and bank cashier's checks drawn for the exact amount, payable to IAT, Ltd, are accepted. Personal checks, certified checks, and cashier's checks cannot be cashed in Freeport. Many insurance policies cover treatment received at the clinic, but the patients themselves are responsible for the successful submission of claims.

Institute of Chronic Disease

416 W. San Ysidro Boulevard, #677
San Ysidro, California 92073
United States

011-526-680-9292

Playas de Tijuana, B.C.
Mexico

011-52-66-30-08-16

Contact Person

Dr. Gustavo Andrade or Alberto Magana.

Primary Personnel

Medical doctor and assistant.

Directions

Patients stay at the San Ysidro Hotel and come to the clinic as outpatients during the morning.

Background

Fifteen years' practice in oncology, nutritional programs in Hospital Contreras (OASIS), former medical director of IAT-West (Burton's Therapy).

Illness Treated

Cancer and immune deficiency disorders.

Treatment Offered

This outpatient clinic treats chronic disease.

Length of Treatment/Stay

Four weeks.

Costs

$4,200.

Method of Payment

Cash, checks, and money orders are accepted.

Instituto Cientifico de Regeneracion, S.A.

Mailing Address:
I.C.D.R. Suite #104
2310 Via Tercero
San Ysidro, California 92073
United States

011-52-66-849231 (Mexico)
Fax: (213) 516-6735

Calle Ensenada #393
Col. Cacho
Tijuana, B.C.
Mexico

011-52-66-849237

Contact Person

Jean Hesse, a former cancer patient of the institute. Write to her at P.O. Box 503, Gardena, California 90247, or phone (213) 538-3277.

Primary Personnel

Neil Norton, M.D. (diagnostic research).

Directions

After crossing the international border, proceed onto bridge under overpass. Remain in right lane while crossing the bridge. Make no left turns. After crossing bridge, turn right at first traffic circle and get into left lane immediately. In a very short distance is another traffic circle. Proceed through this circle without turning, staying to the left. At the first traffic signal turn left. Go one block and turn left again. Continue across a major intersection (Aqua Caliente). Continue up the street (Calle Ensenada) until you reach the institute. It is on your left near the end of the block. It is a large two-story building with a brown cement-block wall on one side of the walkway and a rock wall on the other. At the front of the second story is a large mural. There are no street signs.

Background

Dr. Norton is licensed by the Mexican government. He has been practicing for forty years. The outpatient clinic has what it calls a urine probability analysis, which uses computer instrumentation to obtain information quickly from the processed specimen. The analysis will indicate various pathological problems, their locations, and a comprehensive diagnosis. Also used in diagnosis and treatment are certain heat and electronic procedures, some of which were developed at the institute. A Symcomp computer analysis uses a list of the patient's symptoms and the results of lab tests to produce complex explanations for the primary cause of a patient's illness.

Illness Treated

Cancer, all degenerative conditions, arthritis, herpes, tuberculosis, diabetes, and multiple sclerosis.

Treatment Offered

Intravenous with oral support, intramuscular injections, and whatever other oral medications are indicated by the computer testing. Heat and electronic procedures are also involved.

Related Readings

Audio tapes of Dr. Norton's lectures are available for a fee.

Length of Treatment/Stay

One week of treatment (including testing and consultations), followed by one week of rest. This pattern is repeated as needed.

Costs

Consultation (six months): $150. Lab work (as needed): $250 to $600. Treatment: depends on medication involved, but the daily average is $125. Urine probability analysis: $50 to $75.

Method of Payment

A deposit of $1,000 is required before treatment and lab tests are begun. Any balance is to be paid upon leaving each week. Cash, traveler's, and personal checks are accepted. Most insurance is applicable.

International Center for Medical and Biological Research, Inc.
(Centro International Medico y Biologico de S.A. de C.V.)

Clinic:
670 Calle de Farallon
Playas de Tijuana
Tijuana, B.C.
Mexico

011-52-66-30-18-53

Information, Payments, and Appointments:
4082 Carmel Springs Way
San Diego, California 92130
United States

(619) 481-5284.

Contact Person

Dr. Suzanne Henig (in California).

Primary Personnel

Adamo Herberto Lopez, M.D.; Gerado Bonilla, M.D.; Salvatore Vargas, M.D.; Riccardo Lopez, B.S. (microbiologist); John Majnarich, Ph.D.

Directions

Patients and visitors will be met at the airport in San Diego and taken to hotels and doctors' appointments, free of charge.

Background

The center was founded for the purpose of developing unique alternative pharmaceuticals and methodologies for treating the terminally ill. These include formulations that have demonstrated efficacy against AIDS and various cancers, autoimmune, and genetic diseases. Some of these formulations have been in development for over a decade, and have demonstrated significant efficacy in both *in vitro* and *in vivo* testing, and on patients. The center's AIDS pharmaceuticals are currently in clinical trials in Europe. Although primarily a research group, the center works closely with licensed physician-specialists to make its treatments available to patients on a reasonable cost basis.

Illness Treated

The center's pharmaceuticals have demonstrated a strong efficacy against AIDS, various cancers (including prostate, breast, liver, lung, bone, testicular, melanoma, multiple myeloma, and leukemia), diabetes, epilepsy, radiation, inflammatory diseases, heart disease, asthma, Parkinson's disease, herpes, rheumatoid arthritis, and osteoarthritis.

Treatment Offered

The center offers only its own treatments in the form of vaccines, oral sera, capsules, and pills. It also offers electromagnetic treatment according to Nordstrom and Rife, chelation of heavy metals under hospital conditions, surgery, dentistry, and hospital facilities.

Related Readings

Suppressed Old and Revolutionary New Therapies in the Treatment of Terminal Disease by Suzanne Henig, Ph.D. Aeolian Press, 1996.

The Cancer Microbe by Alan Cantwell, Jr., M.D. Aries Press, 1990.

The center also publishes the *International Journal of Medicine.*

Length of Treatment/Stay

The center likes patients to stay for three weeks. They see the doctor six times a week for treatment, and full blood tests are taken every week. By the time patients return home, the center can tell whether they are beginning remission.

Costs

These costs reflect the full program (three weeks includes all vaccines, doctor's visits, and blood tests). Patients return home with two to three months' supply of either the standard or custom vaccine. Patients stay in a new, air-conditioned luxury hotel for $60 to $65 per night. Three weeks' visit to clinic: $5,000. Standard cancer vaccine: $4,500. Custom vaccine: $7,200. AIDS vaccines are sent to patients and physicians only (under Mexican law, no one is permitted to treat this disease in Mexico). A two months' supply is $5,500. Asthma, Parkinson's disease, herpes, multiple sclerosis, arthritis, CFS: $1,500. Reparative enzyme (oral): $1,500. Heart disease: $4,500. Plastic surgery, liposuction, biopsies, and cancer surgeries are offered. Hospitalization: $150 per day. Registered nurse: $50 per eight hours. Dental work is also available.

Method of Payment

Cash or traveler's checks are accepted. The patient must pay for services in advance. The center helps the patient receive reimbursement by insurance.

International Medical Center

16 de Septiembre #2215
3203-Cd. Juarez
Mexico

011-52-16-16-26-01

United States Office:
1501 Arizona Street 1-E
El Paso, Texas 79902
United States

(800) 621-8924
(915) 543-5621

Contact Person

A packet of information regarding the facility is available upon request by calling the (800) number above.

Primary Personnel

Jaime Narvaez, M.D.; Armine Arjona, M.D.; Francisco Enriquez, administrator.

Directions

Patients use El Paso International Airport, El Paso Greyhound bus station, or Amtrak station, and are transported to and from the clinic. The clinic is located ten minutes from downtown El Paso.

Background

I.M.C. was started as Clinica Paso del Norte, essentially a cancer clinic until September 1989, when H. Ray Evers, M.D., brought all his talents and protocols to the clinic. In addition to cancer, the clinic now treats all forms of chronic degenerative disease.

Illness Treated

Cancer, heart disease, circulatory problems, arthritis, diabetes, amyotrophic lateral sclerosis (Lou Gehrig's disease), chronic fatigue syndrome, Epstein-Barr virus, candidiasis, hypoglycemia, Parkinson's disease, Alzheimer's disease, and most chronic degenerative diseases.

Treatment Offered

Chelation, hyperbaric oxygen, electrotherapy, hydrotherapy, colon therapy, ozone therapy, detoxification, respiratory therapy, physical therapy, acupuncture, shark and bovine cartilage, Koch vaccine, enzyme and nutritional therapy, and immunotherapy.

Related Readings

Forty-Something Forever by Harold and Arline Brecher.
Bypassing Bypass by Elmer Cranton, M.D.
Sharks Don't Get Cancer by Dr. William I. Lane.
The Chelation Way by Dr. Morton Walker.

Length of Treatment/Stay

Three to four weeks is recommended.

Costs

Total cost depends on the treatment recommended, and varies substantially. The approximate cost for cancer averages $3,500 to $4,000 per week; treatment for other diseases averages $3,000 to $3,500. The cost of the immunotherapy depends on the type and number of injections. A three-day detoxification program is available for $700. All prices include room, board, and transportation from El Paso.

Method of Payment

Cash, personal checks, cashier's checks, money orders, Visa, MasterCard, and American Express are all accepted. Payments are due weekly. Most insurance companies will reimburse the patient.

P. Jayalakshmi, M.D.

6366 Sherwood Road
Philadelphia, Pennsylvania 19151
United States

(215) 473-4226

330 Breezewood Road
Lehighton, Pennsylvania 18235
United States

(215) 473-7453

Contact Person

Dr. Jayalakshmi, Dr. Sampathachar.

Primary Personnel

P. Jayalakshmi, M.D.; K.R. Sampathachar, M.D.

Background

The Philadelphia center offers complete services in holistic medicine and Ayurveda as an outpatient facility with some residential possibilities. The Lehighton center is located on a large, peaceful mountain property overlooking the Poconos. This is a residential facility for complete rejuvenation programs that include specially prepared Ayurvedic meals, Pancha Karma, and other specific treatments that can range from a weekend to several weeks.

Illness Treated

All kinds of cancer.

Treatment Offered

Nutrition, oral supplementation, chelation, megavitamins, oxidative therapy, colonics, Pancha Karma Ayurvedic detoxification, visualization, Simonton technique, immune augmentation therapies, and many others.

Related Readings

All books listed by the Cancer Control Society.

Length of Treatment/Stay

Ranges from one week to one month, followed by long-term maintenance.

Costs

Initial consultation: $60. Colonic: $40. Pancha Karma: $200. Simonton visualization: $65.

Method of Payment

Cash, checks, Visa, and MasterCard are accepted. Itemized receipts are given for insurance purposes.

The Kuhnau Center

Lloyd Building
Paseo Tijuana #406
Desp. 104 Secc. Viva Tijuana
Tijuana, B.C.,
Mexico

011-52-66-835151
Fax: 011-52-66-80-11-21

Mailing Address:
P.O. Box 432014
San Ysidro, California 92143
United States

011-52-66-80-11-21 (private)

Contact Person

Wolfram Kuhnau, M.D.; Ignacio Clapes, assistant; Laura Elena Villasenor, secretary.

Primary Personnel

Wolfram Kuhnau, M.D.

Directions

When you cross the border, go into the right lane. In about one minute is the Pueblo Amigo exit. Take this and go to the right, and you will see a brown building (Lloyd Building).

Background

The center's goal is to seek the cause of diseases, not just to treat the symptoms. Dr. Kuhnau has a background in biochemistry and endocrinology, and uses this knowledge as a basis for his treatments.

Illness Treated

All metabolic diseases, including cancer, autoimmune diseases, and genetic diseases.

Treatment Offered

Embryonic shark tissue transplants.

Length of Treatment/Stay

From three days to six months.

Costs

One shot of transplant, $200.

Method of Payment

Cash or checks are accepted. The patient pays the clinic and then submits the bill to the insurance company.

Richard A. Kunin, M.D.

2698 Pacific Avenue
San Francisco, California 94115
United States

(415) 346-2500
Fax: (415) 346-4991

Contact Person

Jadwiga Mosbauer.

Background

Dr. Kunin has worked in orthomolecular medicine since 1970. He is past president of the Orthomolecular Medical Society and founding president of the Society for Orthomolecular Health Medicine. His strategy is to put nutrition first in medical practice.

Illness Treated

General medicine and psychiatry-neurology.

Treatment Offered

Specific nutrient support, dietary balancing for individual, pesticide detoxification, metal chelation, magnetic therapy, DMSO, fatty acids, amino acids, iodide therapy, and hypnosis training.

Related Readings

Meganutrition by Richard A. Kunin, 1980.
Orthomolecular Medicine for Physicians by Abram Hoffer, 1994.

Length of Treatment/Stay

Six months.

Costs

$600 to $2,000 plus lab.

Method of Payment

Cash, checks, Visa, and MasterCard are accepted. The office assists the patient in filing insurance.

Livingston Foundation Medical Center

3232 Duke Street
San Diego, California 92110
United States

(619) 224-3515
Fax: (619) 224-6253

Contact Person

Patricia Huntley, director.

Primary Personnel

Kenneth C. Forror, M.D.

Directions

Exit Sea World off ramp from Highway 5, or take Rosecrans to Midway and Duke Street.

Background

Livingston Foundation Medical Center was established in 1971 by the late Virginia C. Livingston, M.D., an internationally recognized clinician, healer, and medical researcher who devoted her life to the study of the body's immune system and its relationship to human diseases. Today, the center provides the latest immunological treatment programs based upon the models developed by Dr. Livingston during her more than fifty years of research. The center is staffed by licensed, highly committed, and specially trained physicians, assisted by a complete staff of skilled nurses, laboratory technicians, a nutritionist, and other key support personnel. Livingston Foundation Medical Center has successfully treated thousands of patients from around the world.

Illness Treated

Immune deficiency diseases such as allergies, arthritis, cancer, lupus, and scleroderma.

Treatment Offered

Two treatment programs are offered. The ten-day comprehensive program strengthens the body's immune system, using natural, nontoxic, noninvasive methods, so that it may effectively fight disease. This program integrates vaccines, nutrition, and dietary supplementation, along with psychological education and counseling in stress management, relaxation, and visualization techniques. A two-day prevention program is also offered for those who wish to maintain optimum health.

Related Readings

Food Alive (a cookbook).

Conquest of Cancer: Vaccines and Diet by Virginia Livingston-Wheeler, M.D., with Edmond G. Addeo. Franklin Watts Publishing, 1984. (Patients are encouraged to read this before going for treatments.)

Cancer, A New Breakthrough by Virginia Livingston-Wheeler, M.D.

Compendium by Virginia Livingston-Wheeler, M.D. Reprints of Dr. Livingston's published papers and scientific articles.

These books may be ordered through the medical center.

Length of Treatment/Stay

Ten days (Monday to Friday for two consecutive weeks).

Costs

Initial consultation for new patients is free. The estimated cost of the full treatment program is $5,500 for ten days. The estimated cost of the preventive program is $1,200. Living expenses are not included. A detailed information packet is available upon request.

Method of Payment

Insurance may or may not cover fees, for which the patients are financially responsible. Cash, personal checks, traveler's checks, money orders, MasterCard, and Visa are accepted.

Lost Horizon Health Awareness Center

P.O. Box 620550
Oviedo, Florida 32762-0550
United States

(407) 365-6681
Fax: (407) 365-1834

Contact Person

Roy B. Kupsinel, M.D.

Primary Personnel

Roy B. Kupsinel, M.D.

Directions

From I-4, exit at Longwood, Florida, and proceed east on Highway 434 for twelve miles to Shangri-La Lane. Or: Exit Greeneway at Highway 434, and proceed east for one-eighth of a mile to Shangri-La Lane.

Background

Dr. Kupsinel's approach is holistic. He deals with the entire being: physical, mental, emotional, and spiritual. His emphasis is not on treating the disease but on treating the person who may have various health problems.

Illness Treated

Degenerative diseases.

Treatment Offered

EDTA chelation therapy, preventive medicine, nutrition, diet, supplements, positive thinking, exercise, and other modalities.

Costs

Costs were not submitted for publication.

Magaziner Medical Center

1907 Greentree Road
Cherry Hill, New Jersey 08003
United States

(609) 424-8222
Fax: (609) 424-2599

Contact Person

Allan Magaziner, D.O., P.C.

Primary Personnel

Allan Magaziner, D.O., P.C.

Directions

Two miles from Exit 4 of the New Jersey Turnpike. One block from Route 70. One mile from Route 73.

Background

The focus is on nontoxic treatments utilizing natural therapies to enhance human functioning and to prevent disease. Treatments include oral and intravenous therapies, diet changes, and lifestyle modifications.

Illness Treated

Prostate, breast, lung, and bowel cancer; Alzheimer's disease; multiple sclerosis; atherosclerosis; cardiovascular disease; cerebral vascular disease/strokes; allergies; arthritis; asthma; hypertension; chronic fatigue syndrome; premenstrual syndrome; chemical sensitivities; migraine; and heavy metal toxicity.

Treatment Offered

Oral and intravenous vitamins; minerals; amino acids; oral botanicals; herbs; enzymes; homeopathics; chelation therapy; removal of toxic metals; and detoxification.

Length of Treatment/Stay

Varies, depending on treatment.

Costs

Varies, depending on treatment.

Method of Payment

Cash, checks, Visa, and MasterCard are accepted. Insurance is not accepted.

Mantell Medical Clinic

General and Family Practice
6505 Mars Road
Cranberry Township, Pennsylvania 16066-5109
United States

(412) 776-5610

Contact Person

Patricia Bartonas, office manager.

Primary Personnel

Donald Mantell, M.D.; John Lanurn, L.P.N.; Evelyn Mancell, colonics therapist; Armon Croll, electroacupuncturist.

Directions

Pennsylvania Turnpike Exit 3 (north from Pittsburgh; south from Ohio) to Route 19. North to first light. Right on Route 228. Left onto Dutilh Road. Make first right onto Mars Road.

Background

The facilities are two converted ranch houses with two floors and an extensive parking area.

Illness Treated

Cancer, arthritis, allergies, multiple sclerosis, asthma, and musculoskeletal pains.

Treatment Offered

A multifaceted metabolic approach. The major elements of the therapy are: diet, vitamins, minerals, enzymes, herbs, homeopathy, and an IV with DMSO and vitamin C. Ancillary treatments include colonic irrigation, electroacupuncture, chelation, clinical ecology, and neural therapy (for pain).

Related Readings

Crackdown on Cancer With Good Nutrition by Ruth Yale Long. Nutrition Education Association, 1983.

You Don't Have to Die by Harry M. Hoxsey. Joseph C. Carl, 1977.

The Cancer Syndrome by Ralph W. Moss. Grove Press, 1980.

"Colon Hydrotherapy." *The Nutritional Consultant*, May 1986.

DMSO Handbook by Dr. Bruce Halstead.

The Death of Cancer by Harold W. Manner. Advanced Century Publishing, 1978.

Length of Treatment/Stay

This is an outpatient clinic. The patient will have to stay in a motel if from out of town. Intensive treatments at the clinic run from two to four weeks, depending on the severity of the case.

Costs

The first visit costs $350. Of that, $95 is billed to the patient's insurance (if there is appropriate coverage) and $255 is due. The second visit costs $65 plus supplements (one month's supply ranges from $400 to $650). This doesn't include ancillary treatments.

Method of Payment

Cash, checks, MasterCard, and Visa are accepted. Insurance covers diagnostic testing only. Out-of-state residents must pay for diagnostic testing unless covered by Medicare or Blue Shield.

Edward W. McDonagh, D.O.
Charles J. Rudolph, D.O., Ph.D.

2800-A Kendallwood Parkway
Gladstone, Missouri 64119
United States

(816) 453-5940
Fax: (816) 453-1140

Contact Person

Charles J. Rudolph, D.O., Ph.D.

Primary Personnel

Twenty-two employees.

Directions

Gladstone is a northern suburb of Kansas City. The clinic is about two miles north of I-35, Antioch exit in N. Kansas City.

Illness Treated

Heart disease, arthritis, fatigue, allergies, and candida.

Treatment Offered

Chelation therapy, nutrition, and general practice.

Related Readings

Chelation Can Cure by Edward W. McDonagh.

Length of Treatment/Stay

Initially, three to six months.

Costs

$2,000 to $4,000, depending on the severity and length of treatment.

Method of Payment

Cash, check, Discover, MasterCard, and Visa are accepted.

The McDougall Program at St. Helena Hospital

650 Sanatarium Road
Deer Park, California 94576
United States

(707) 963-6365

Contact Person

Birgitta Karlman.

Primary Personnel

John McDougall, M.D., medical director and founder.

Directions

One and one half hours north of San Francisco. Take I-80 to 37 to 29 to St. Helena.

Background

The program involves a starch-based diet with fresh fruits and vegetables, exercise, psychological comfort, and spiritual strength. The program has cared for over 1,300 people over ten years.

Illness Treated

Cardiovascular disease such as angina and high blood pressure, adult diabetes, arthritis, multiple sclerosis, colitis, chronic indigestion, obesity, food allergies, nephritis, and mild chronic kidney failure.

Treatment Offered

The program combines diet and exercise with medical treatments (used as second line therapies).

Related Readings

The McDougall Plan by John McDougall, M.D.
McDougall's Medicine by John McDougall, M.D.
The McDougall Program—12 Days to Dynamic Health by John McDougall, M.D.
The McDougall Program for a Healthy Heart by John McDougall, M.D.
The New McDougall Cookbook by John McDougall, M.D.

Length of Treatment/Stay

Twelve days.

Costs

Approximately $4,000, plus a reduced rate for companion.

Method of Payment

Cash, checks, and Visa are accepted. Most of the medical care is covered by insurance companies.

Thomas McNaughton, M.D.

1521 Dolphin Street
Sarasota, Florida 34236
United States

(813) 365-6273

Contact Person

Kari Schulman, office manager.

Primary Personnel

Kari Schulman, office manager; Charlotte Currie, receptionist.

Background

M.D., Indiana University School of Medicine, 1966. Member, American College of Advancement in Medicine (ACAM); American Holistic Medical Association; American Preventive Medicine Association; National Center for Homeopathy; National Health Federation; International Bio-Oxidative Medicine Foundation; Complementary Medical Association (founder).

Illness Treated

Chronic degenerative diseases, chronic fatigue syndrome, environmental illness, immune dysregulation, cardiac/pulmonary diseases, and irritable bowel syndrome.

Treatment Offered

Chelation therapy, bio-oxidative therapy, nutritional medicine, and immune system enhancement.

Costs

Not submitted for publication.

Method of Payment

Checks, cash, Visa, MasterCard, and Discover are accepted.

Metabolic Associates

195 Columbia Turnpike
Florham, New Jersey 07932
United States

(201) 377-7300

Contact Person

Lisa Haverstick, R.D.

Primary Personnel

Michael Rothkopf, M.D., F.A.C.P.; Kenneth Storch, M.D., Ph.D.

Background

Drs. Rothkopf and Storch are internists and board-certified nutritionists. They offer a nutritional approach to treating various diseases, as an addition to whatever conventional or alternative treatment the patient may receive from his or her regular doctor.

Illness Treated

Any disease with a nutritional component, including cancer, AIDS, high cholesterol, and obesity.

Treatment Offered

Nutrition and cancer prevention, diet modification, and nutritional support.

Length of Treatment/Stay

Varies, depending on the individual case.

Costs

An initial consultation costs $250 to $275. Follow-up visits are less, but the amount depends on the individual case.

Method of Payment

Cash, checks, credit cards, and insurance are accepted.

Mission Medical Clinic

Tijuana, B.C.
Mexico

(619) 662-1578 (U.S.A.)

Mailing Address:
4492 Camino de la Plaza
Suite 362
San Ysidro, California 92173
United States

Primary Personnel

James Gunier, H.M.D., Ph.D.; Roberto Diaz, M.D., Ph.D.; N. Osuna, M.D.

Directions

Approximately fifteen miles south of San Diego. Call for exact directions.
Transportation is provided to and from the clinic.

Background

Founded in 1983, the clinic is world-famous for its tumor and cancer therapy program.
It claims that tumors decrease very rapidly during this program. Thousands have
regained their health, strength, and vitality.

Illness Treated

All forms of cancer: breast, skin, ovarian, prostate, stomach, intestine, colon, liver, lung,
bone, leukemia, brain, mouth, throat, uterus, rectum. Also: AIDS, arthritis,
Alzheimer's, stroke, paralysis, rare neurological diseases, chronic degenerative diseases, and age-related problems.

Treatment Offered

Nontoxic therapies: tumor reduction therapy, tumorin, therapeutic immunology, RNA
regeneration, Koch, Ridasa, immune therapy, rare homeopathic tumor remedies, HCL
mineral chloride infusion, super IV drips, herbology, Rife, Dia-Pulse, poultices, counseling, diet, lifestyle changes, and a personalized follow-up program. The clinic also
uses European anti-aging live cell revitalization injections to strengthen and support
the immune system.

Related Readings

The center will furnish an information packet and testimonials upon request.

Length of Treatment/Stay

Two to three weeks of treatment is recommended.

Costs

Treatment: $150 to $600 per day, depending on which program the patient chooses.

Method of Payment

Traveler's checks are accepted. Most private insurance companies will cover at least a considerable portion of the expenses.

Robert Nagourney, M.D.

Rational Therapeutics
3601 Elm Avenue
Long Beach, California 90807
United States

(310) 426-8903
(310) 427-3052

Contact Person

Steven Evans, M.A., or Robert Salti.

Primary Personnel

Research and clinical staff.

Directions

Located at Elm and 36th Street in Long Beach, at the junction of the 405 and 710 freeways.

Background

Board-certified hematologist and oncologist.

Illness Treated

Blood disorders and solid tumors.

Treatment Offered

Laboratory-based therapy utilizing short form (apoptotic) assays to identify active agents and eliminate inactive agents.

Length of Treatment/Stay
Variable.

Costs
$500 to $2,500.

Method of Payment
Insurance covers most evaluations. Other than that, methods of payment are variable.

Natural Medicine Clinic

213 Hywood Lane
Bolingbrook, Illinois 60440
United States
(630) 378-0610

Primary Personnel
Dr. J. Steven Holcomb, director.

Directions
Four lights west of I-355 and Boughton. Six lights north of Stevenson (55).

Illness Treated
Any illness, including cancer, when natural medicine is preferred by the patient.

Treatment Offered
Nutritional medicine, herbal medicine, qi gong (chee kung), and acupuncture.

Related Readings
Textbook of Natural Medicine by Murray, et. al.
The Practice of Chinese Medicine by Maciocia.
Breast Cancer: What You Should Know by Austin.
Natural Alternatives to OTCA Prescription by Murray.
Alternative Medicine—The Definitive Guide by Goldberg.

Length of Treatment/Stay
Six to nine months, depending on the patient.

Costs

$200 to $500 per month, depending on the patient's condition, the strength of the patient's constitution, the duration of the patient's condition, and individual goals.

Method of Payment

Cash, checks, Visa, MasterCard, and some insurance are accepted. The clinic accepts most 80:20 plans after the first visit.

Nevada Clinic

3720 Howard Hughes Parkway
Suite 270
Las Vegas, Nevada 89109
United States

(702) 732-1400
(800) 641-6661

Contact Person

Larry L. Woolf, clinic administrator.

Primary Personnel

F. Fuller Royal, M.D., H.M.D., medical director; Daniel F. Royal, D.O., H.M.D.

Directions

Located one-and-a-half miles north of McCarran International Airport, the clinic is at the northwest corner of Sands and Paradise.

Background

A staff of twenty runs this 7,000-square-foot outpatient clinic. The staff performs routine blood tests and standard procedures done by other physicians, as well as nonstandard procedures. The clinic has electrodiagnostic equipment for measuring abnormal electro-magnetic energy fields of the body.

Illness Treated

Cancer; the best responders are liver metastases and colon and breast cancers. Also allergies, arthritis (all types), lupus erythematosus and other collagen diseases, cardiovascular diseases, arteriosclerotic diseases, and AIDS.

Treatment Offered

Homeopathy, chelation, acupuncture, and acuscope.

Length of Treatment/Stay

One to fourteen days. Thirty days for chelation patients.

Costs

The cost for a new patient is $900 to $1,200, which covers the cost of complete evaluation, allergy testing, medication, and treatment for the first day. Return office visits are $60 each day.

Method of Payment

Cash, checks, Visa, MasterCard, and Discover are accepted. The clinic will not accept insurance.

New Hope Medical Center

411 Andrews Road, Suite 420
Durham, North Carolina 27705
United States

(919) 382-0777

Contact Person

Naima Abdel-Ghany, M.D.

Background

Preventive therapy, internal medicine, immunotherapy, complementary therapy, and nutritional therapy.

Illness Treated

Cancer, heart disease, arthritis, and other chronic diseases.

Treatment Offered

Nutritional counseling, chelation therapy, and bio-oxidative therapy.

Length of Treatment/Stay

One week to three months.

Costs

Initial consultation $160. Office visits $35 to $100. Cost of tests varies.

Method of Payment

Insurance and self-payment are accepted.

Northern Health Inc.

P.O. Box 200
Glencairn, Ontario L0M 1KO
Canada

(705) 466-2015
Fax: (705) 466-2774

Contact Person

Rudolf E. Falk, M.D.

Primary Personnel

Rudolf E. Falk, M.D.

Background

The clinic is dedicated to the development of innovative therapies for the increasing number of cancer patients, many of whom are unresponsive to standard cancer treatment. Dr. Falk founded the Goldie Rotman Cancer Clinic in 1978 and the Falk Oncology Centre in 1986. The Falk Oncology Centre was the first private cancer clinic in Canada. In January 1996 the centre was moved seventy miles north of Toronto and was renamed Northern Health Inc. Dr. Falk has had thirty years of experience in treating cancer and until a few years ago, ran a productive basic laboratory at the University of Toronto, where he is Professor of Surgery. Dr. Falk is also a consultant at the multidisciplinary Americas Research and Treatment Centre in Santo Domingo, Dominican Republic.

Illness Treated

Primarily cancer, but also arterial disease.

Treatment Offered

Patients are treated with a combination of drugs, including low-dose chemotherapy, nonsteroidal anti-inflammatory drugs (NSAIDs), and high doses of vitamin C, all of which are combined with hyaluronic acid (hyaluronan, HA), which is a targeting carrier molecule. The use of hyaluronic acid allows for better penetration of the drug to the tumor, and also better targeting, so the severe side effects of drugs are not felt. On occasion, hyperthermia is used, as well.

Length of Treatment/Stay
Three to four days approximately once per month.

Costs
$900 to $1,800 per day of treatment. Actual cost depends on the type of tumor, previous treatment, and extent of disease.

Method of Payment
Checks, cash, Visa, American Express, and MasterCard are accepted. Most major insurance companies cover costs.

Oasis Hospital
(formerly Hospital Ernesto Contreras)

Paseo Playas #19
Playas de Tijuana, B.C. 22700
Mexico

011-526-680-1850
Fax: 011-526-680-1952

Mailing Address:
P.O. Box 439045
San Ysidro, California 92143
United States

(800) 700-1850
Fax: (619) 297-3242

Contact Person
Call Lisa Elder at the 800 number for general information about the hospital. She will have one of the doctors call you for any medical information.

Primary Personnel
Dr. Ernesto Contreras Sr., general director and founder; Dr. Ernesto Contreras Jr., medical director and oncologist; Dr. Francisco Contreras, general administrator and surgeon.

Directions

If you are driving, after crossing the border take the lane with the sign "Rosarito, Ensenada." Follow it without changing lanes. After several turns it will lead you to Rosarita, Ensenada Toll Road and Playas de Tijuana. Drive west about six miles. When you get close to the ocean, take the right lane, which goes to the beach (playas). Half a mile farther, you will see the big bull ring. Across the street is Oasis Hospital. All patients must have a reservation in advance.

Background

Dr. Ernesto Contreras Sr. has completed fifty-five years of medical practice. He has devoted thirty-three years to finding less aggressive but more effective alternatives for the treatment of cancer and other degenerative diseases. He is assisted by his two sons, who are medical doctors and cancer specialists, and by twenty-five other specialists and health care professionals. Facilities include a fifty-bed hospital, outpatient accommodations, a pharmacy, a twenty-four-hour clinical laboratory, a complete radiology department, Direx Lithotripsy machine, and a cafeteria that serves the special diets that patients require. Oasis Hospital is the largest comprehensive cancer treatment center in northwestern Mexico.

Illness Treated

Cancer; also most chronic degenerative diseases, such as arthritis, multiple sclerosis, and lupus.

Treatment Offered

Metabolic therapy, using amygdalin (laetrile), shark cartilage, enzymes, and megadoses of vitamins A and C; immune therapy; and Warburg therapy, using a formula developed by Dr. Cone. All the programs are nontoxic and use a special diet, detoxification, and immunemodulators. Part of the therapy involves the use of psychological and spiritual methods to build up the immune system. English services are offered to the patients and their companions on Sundays from 10 a.m. to noon. Dr. Contreras Sr. also conducts Bible studies and sing-alongs. Also offered is a cancer prevention program that includes the Arthur (AMID) test.

Related Readings

Amygdalin, a Monographic Study. Kem S.A. Laboratories.

Length of Treatment/Stay

The average is three to four weeks.

Costs

Costs will depend on the treatment or treatments for your particular case. Lisa Elder can quote all costs and discuss method of payment and insurance.

Ozone Research Center
(Centro Nacional de Investigaciones del Ozono)

Ave. 15 y calle 230, Siboney, Playa
P.O. Box 6880
Havana
Cuba

011-53-7-21-05-88
011-53-7-21-01-22
Fax: 011-53-7-33-04-97
Fax: 011-53-7-21-02-33

E-mail: ozono@infomed.sld.cu

Primary Personnel

Carlos Hernandez Castro, Ph.D., director.

Directions

Havana is accessible by plane.

Background

Ozone Research Center is a scientific institution devoted to research, development, and applications of ozone. Its senior staff has been involved in this work since 1972. In the medical field, work started in 1985, and the main directions are: development of ozone therapy procedures for the treatment of different diseases (these procedures are now extensively employed in the main hospitals and health centers of Cuba); synthesis and application of ozonated substances in medicine; and design and production of ozonizers for therapeutic purposes. These lines are supported by basic research on mechanisms of ozone action on living organisms, and by experimental work from laboratory *in vitro* and preclinical studies to controlled clinical trials. Ozone therapy is a versatile therapeutic approach, simple to perform, and effective in the treatment of different diseases. It induces an improvement in oxygen metabolism; an immunemodulation effect; and a protective action against oxygen reactive species, which are responsible for several organic disorders.

Illness Treated

Chronic degenerative diseases, such as senile dementia, Parkinson's disease, arthritis, diabetic neuroangiopathy, glaucoma, and cancers. Other pathologies not included here could be submitted for consideration.

Treatment Offered

Personalized treatments are based on ozone therapy procedures, which can be administered in different ways, according to the pathology and the state of the patient.

Length of Treatment/Stay

Treatments usually take three to five weeks, depending on the pathology and the state of the patient.

Costs

Not submitted for publication.

Method of Payment

Cash or credit cards without transfer from U.S. branches are accepted.

Pacific Center for Naturopathic Medicine

1919 Broadway, Suite 206
Bellingham, Washington 98225
United States

(360) 734-0045

2209 West Broadway
Vancouver, B.C. V6K 2E4
Canada

(604) 734-0244

Primary Personnel

Rachelle Herdman, N.D., M.D.

Directions

To Bellingham: Ninety minutes north of Seattle; use the Bellingham or Seattle airport, or take Interstate 5, Exit 256, Meridian Street westbound. Turn right onto Broadway. To Vancouver: Twenty minutes from Vancouver airport, and accessible by bus. Located in the Kitsilano district, one block west of the Broadway-Arbutus Street intersection.

Background

The center's naturopathic medicine programs integrate medical arts and sciences; care for the whole person, body and psyche; attend to the underlying causes of illness; and use only natural remedies. Recognizing illness as a personal journey, all aspects are explored via conventional diagnostic testing, Asian medicine assessment, and supportive personal counseling. Treatments may emphasize physical, metabolic, mental, and/or spiritual dimensions, according to individual need and interest. Dr. Herdman was previously a pathologist at London University in England. Deeply committed to natural medicine, she went on to receive a doctorate in Naturopathy from Bastyr University in Seattle, and now practices exclusively naturopathic medicine. She also speaks locally and internationally.

Illness Treated

All chronic problems including cancer; autoimmune, neurological, cardiovascular, and digestive disorders; chronic fatigue; and depression.

Treatment Offered

Nutritional medicine, including a diet of whole, natural foods tailored for diagnosis, body type, focality, and season; Chinese five elements and Ayurveda; carefully-selected supplements; cooking classes; lifestyle and exercise guidance; homeopathy; mind-body medicine—in-depth and Jungian counseling, dreams, drawing, journaling, and visualization—to consider the meanings and impact of illness; and botanical medicine, including individualized prescriptions of herbal tinctures, botanical teas, and plant extracts.

Length of Treatment/Stay

Series of one-hour medical consultations with Dr. Herdman. Cooking classes: series of four-hour participatory sessions for one to ten people. Five-day intensives including all facets of treatment and lifestyle change (maximum five people).

Costs

As of 1997 (U.S. or Canadian dollars, according to locations): One-hour office visit, $90; four-hour cooking class, $85; five-day intensive, $2,000; remedies (estimated range), $10 to $300.

Method of Payment

Cash or checks are accepted.

Panama City Clinic
(formerly Akbar Clinic)

340 West 23rd Street
Suite E
Panama City, Florida 32405
United States

(904) 763-7689
Fax: (904) 763-5396

Primary Personnel

Naima Abdel-Ghany, M.D.

Directions

The clinic is located on the coast of the Gulf of Mexico. Three airlines connect Panama City Airport with all major cities of the United States and the world.

Background

The clinic offers conventional medical services in addition to the multimodality immunotherapy program, which is a unique, comprehensive nontoxic metabolic therapy designed to enhance or restore the body's immune system. The protocol is based in part on the work of Dr. Josef Issels. It is useful in the treatment of conditions associated with immune deficiency. The clinic is a multispecialty ambulatory medical facility. Arrangements can be made for any number of patients. Five languages are spoken there: English, French, Spanish, German, and Arabic.

Illness Treated

All illnesses, including cancer, AIDS, and chronic degenerative diseases associated with an immune deficiency.

Treatment Offered

The multimodality immunotherapy program is a nontoxic metabolic treatment with virtually no side effects. It includes nutritional adjustment; nutritional supplementation with certain vitamins, minerals, and enzymes; several natural immune enhancers; acupuncture; hyperpyrexia (fever therapy); and a comprehensive stress reduction program utilizing specialized counseling and biofeedback training. Adequate oxygenation and elimination of toxic metabolic waste products is maintained. A graded physical exercise program is designed to suit the patient's tolerance. Any existing focus of chronic infection is treated, if applicable. Additional treatment modalities may be used according to the patient's condition. A comprehensive assessment of the immune functions is carried out prior to, and at intervals during, the treatment, in order to monitor the patient's response to the therapy. Other diagnostic studies are obtained as the condition may require.

Related Readings

Immunotherapy in Progressive Metastatic Cancer by J. Issels, M.D.

Effect of Nigella Sativa (The Black Seed) and Immunity by A. Elkadi, M.D., and O. Kandil.

Garlic and the Immune System in Humans: Its Effect on Natural Killer Cells by A. Elkadi, M.D., and O. Kandil.

Length of Treatment/Stay

The intensive program is given for two to three months, during which the patient must be present at the clinic. This is followed by a home maintenance program, which may have to be followed indefinitely. In some situations, an intensive booster program, for a shorter period of time, may be needed on a yearly basis.

Costs

The initial consultation costs $160. Other fees depend on the treatment given. The clinic is an outpatient facility, but accommodations are available in the vicinity.

Method of Payment

Some of the medical services are covered by the majority of insurance companies. The clinic staff will be happy to assist the patient in the preparation of insurance forms, if needed.

Partners in Wellness

375 Glensprings Drive, Suite 400
Cincinnati, Ohio 45246
United States

(513) 851-8790

Contact Person

Dr. Nelly Macheret.

Primary Personnel

Leonid Macheret, M.D., director; Phyllis Walker.

Illness Treated

Arthritis, cardiovascular disorders, chronic fatigue syndrome, allergies, degenerative disease, diabetes, metabolic diseases, hypoglycemia, obesity, anxiety, skin disorders, fibromyalgia, and back pain.

Treatment Offered

Preventive medicine, chelation therapy, general practice, acupuncture therapy, osteopathic manipulation, orthomolecular medicine, nutritional supplementation, weight reduction and weight management, stress management, yoga, ethnic herbs, and Ayurvedic remedies.

Related Readings

Bypassing the Bypass.
Forty-Something Forever by Harold and Arline Brecher.

The Medical Miracles by Douglas Campbell, M.D.
Sharks Don't Get Cancer by Dr. I. William Lane and Linda Comac.
Shark Cartilage by Dr. Duarte.

Length of Treatment/Stay
Individualized program for each client.

Costs
Cost analysis is calculated for each client depending on the type of treatment administered for their program.

Method of Payment
Cash, checks, Visa, MasterCard, and Discovery are accepted.

Perlmutter Health Center
720 Goodlette Road North, #203
Naples, Florida 34102
United States

(941) 649-7400
Internet: http://www.perlhealth.com

Contact Person
Fran Lankford.

Primary Personnel
David Perlmutter, M.D., director; Myron Lezak, M.D.

Directions
From I-75, Exit 16 (Pine Ridge Road) west to Goodlette Road. Turn left and head south to 7th Avenue North. Turn left at the light and go to stop sign. Turn left and follow road around the lake to the 800 building. From U.S. 41, turn left at 7th Avenue North (about one mile south of Coastland Mall). Go past two traffic lights. At stop sign, turn left and go around the lake to the 800 building.

Background
With fifteen years of experience in the practice of medicine, Dr. Perlmutter founded the Perlmutter Health Center to provide a unique complementary approach to a wide vari-

ety of health-related problems and preventive medical care. The center offers state-of-the-art laboratory techniques combined with more traditional approaches, including vitamin and nutritional therapies.

Illness Treated

The center deals with a variety of medical problems, including arthritis; elevated cholesterol; bowel and digestive disorders; obesity; cardiovascular problems; respiratory disorders, including asthma; various pain syndromes; low back and neck disorders; chronic fatigue syndrome; allergies; fibromyalgia; environmental sensitivity; cancer; and many other illnesses. Dr. Perlmutter is a board-certified neurologist, and the approach offered at the center is particularly well-suited to neurological problems, including headache; epilepsy; stroke; parkinsonism; dementia (including Alzheimer's disease); myasthenia gravis; multiple sclerosis; amyotrophic lateral sclerosis; dystonia; other movement disorders; and neuropathy.

Treatment Offered

The approach offered by the Perlmutter Health Center recognizes the importance of the advances of modern medicine and utilizes these techniques fully. In addition, Dr. Perlmutter and his staff rely upon a variety of complementary health techniques, including vitamin therapy, nutritional supplementation, herbal preparations, massage therapy, EDTA chelation therapy, and others, to provide a comprehensive, fully integrated treatment plan specifically designed for the needs of the individual.

Related Readings

LifeGuide: Your Guide to a Longer and Healthier Life by David Perlmutter, M.D. LifeGuide Press Publishers, Naples, Florida.

Length of Treatment/Stay

Average two to four weeks, but the programs learned are continued lifelong.

Costs

Initial evaluation is $285. Further costs depend upon the patient's needs. The center is happy to assist out-of-town patients with local accommodations, with special rates available at several local hotels.

Method of Payment

Cash, checks, Visa, and MasterCard are accepted. The center submits applications for Medicare participants.

William H. Philpott, M.D.

P.O. Box 50655
Midwest City, Oklahoma 73140
United States

(405) 390-1444
Fax: (405) 390-2968

Background

This is an F.D.A.-approved research project on the possible benefits of magnetic resonance bio-oxidative therapy.

Illness Treated

The Bio-Electro-Magnetic Institute is researching the value of magnets in areas such as
pain relief, sleep enhancement, reversal of atherosclerosis, detoxification, mental and
emotional problems, and several chronic, degenerative diseases.

Treatment Offered

Magnetic therapy. A local physician provides Dr. Philpott with an initial statement of
the research subject's condition prior to magnetic therapy. After receiving this initial
statement, Dr. Philpott prepares a magnetic research protocol to be followed. The local
research monitoring physician makes the initial report and additional reports to Dr.
Philpott at four-month intervals. If needed, arrangements can be made to be evaluated
and monitored by a physician in Oklahoma, with Dr. Philpott as a consultant.

Related Readings

Magnetic Therapy Newsletter by William H. Philpott, M.D.
Cancer: The Magnetic/Oxygen Answer by William H. Philpott, M.D.
Magnetic Therapy for Rheumatoid Arthritis by William H. Philpott, M.D.

Length of Treatment/Stay

Variable.

Costs

For this consultation service of the research protocol, the initial and periodic communication with the monitoring physician and research subject, there is a fee of $150
paid by the research subject to William H. Philpott, M.D. The patient pays the physician and buys the magnets. Insurance companies and Medicare will not pay for magnetic resonance bio-oxidative therapy until its values are scientifically and ethically
established.

Preventive Medical Center of Marin, Inc.

25 Mitchell Boulevard, Suite 8
San Rafael, California 94903
United States

(415) 472-2343
Fax: (415) 472-7636

Contact Person

Lora Pascucci.

Primary Personnel

Elson M. Haas, M.D.

Background

Created in 1984, Preventive Medical Center of Marin (PMCM) is a continually evolving, integrated health care facility, which provides a medical multidisciplinary approach to health problems, bridging Western medicine with lifestyle counseling and a focus on natural therapies.

Illness Treated

PMCM is a general family practice, treating all kinds of medical problems, both acute and chronic illnesses, with a wide range of therapies. The center uses a three-level approach to therapy and prevention of further problems—lifestyle change, natural therapies, and pharmaceutical treatment. There is a focus upon preventive medicine, particularly for cardiovascular disease and cancer, as well as general health assessment from a medical and functional medicine point of view. Medical concerns commonly treated at PMCM include gastrointestinal concerns, yeast (candida) and parasites, viral diseases, musculoskeletal problems, and pain disorders.

Treatment Offered

The treatment programs for most medical/health concerns are multidisciplinary, unless the patient requests or expects a certain modality. A key focus is to help each individual understand the origins of his or her concerns, and to educate and inform the patient about the treatment modalities. Then together, as a collaborative process, decisions are made regarding the appropriate treatment regimen specific to the medical concern and the individual belief and desire of each person. Treatments include nutritional and herbal therapies, detoxification practices, osteopathy and manipulation, acupuncture and Chinese herbal therapy, bodywork, and psychotherapy.

Related Readings

The Detox Diet: The How-To Guide for Cleansing the Body From Toxic Substances by Elson M. Haas, M.D.

A Diet for All Seasons by Elson M. Haas, M.D.

Staying Healthy With Nutrition: The Complete Guide to Diet and Nutritional Medicine by Elson M. Haas, M.D.

Staying Healthy With the Seasons by Elson M. Haas, M.D.

Smart Medicine for a Healthier Child: A Practical A-to-Z Reference to Natural and Conventional Treatments for Infants & Children by Janet Zand, Rachel Walton, and Bob Rountree, M.D.

The Wisdom Within by Dr. Irving and Susan Oyle.

Length of Treatment/Stay

Length of time is totally individual; however, the focus of PMCM is to evaluate, educate, help heal, and send patients back into their lives having learned how to be their own doctors, at least more so than when they first came to the center.

Costs

Costs vary depending on testing and length of treatments. First consultations range from $95 to $175, depending on the time and involvement. Lab costs may vary from $50 to $1,000, depending on degree of investigation. The center offers a wide array of basic medical as well as innovative and functional testing. Individual programs are created with each patient based on his or her budget and desire.

Method of Payment

The center accepts MasterCard, Visa, and ATMs. Much of its services are covered by third-party insurance. Payment is expected at the time of service unless the center is contracted with your insurance company. The center is a Medicare provider as well as a member of many PPO programs; these plans are billed directly for visits and laboratory testing.

James R. Privitera, M.D.

105 North Grandview Avenue
Covina, California 91723
United States

(818) 966-1618
Fax: (818) 966-7226

Contact Person

Any of the office staff.

Directions

Phone for directions. The office is about twenty miles east of Los Angeles.

Background

This nutrition and allergy office treats the whole body with vitamins and food supplements. It performs routine tests including a darkfield, a mineral analysis, and a urine indican, so that the doctor can give the patients the best recommendation possible.

Illness Treated

The doctor sees patients with all sorts of illnesses, including arthritis, cancer, chronic fatigue, premenstrual syndrome, and circulatory problems, and also patients who are seeking to stay as healthy as possible.

Treatment Offered

Nutritional and immunological enhancement. The staff also performs chelation therapy. Dr. Privitera has done extensive work with the darkfield microscope.

Related Readings

Dr. Privitera has written many articles on nutrition, and will soon have a book out on clotting.

Length of Treatment/Stay

This is an outpatient facility. Some of its cancer patients receive nutritional IV's, which take approximately two hours per treatment.

Costs

Please phone for prices, as costs vary.

Method of Payment

Checks, cash, Visa, and MasterCard are accepted. Insurance is not accepted.

Program for Studies of Alternative Medicines
(Programa de Estudios de Medicinas Alternativas)

Centro Universitario de los Altos
Universidad de Guadalajara
Carretera a Yahualica KM. 7
Tepatitlan, Jal.
Mexico

011-378-13532; 011-378-15133; 011-378-15134.
Private practice numbers: 011-36-377237; 011-36-515476.
Fax: 011-36-370030 or 011-36-193722
E-mail: hsolorza@udgserv.cencar.udg.mx

Primary Personnel

Hector E. Solorzano, M.D., Ph.D., director.

Directions

Guadalajara, the second largest city in Mexico, is accessible by plane, car, and train.

Background

The University of Guadalajara's Program for Studies of Alternative Medicines was established in 1985. Its goal is to investigate, teach, and spread the qualified use of alternative medicines. A seminar is usually held each month on a particular alternative medicine. Some of the seminars are for lay people who want to learn how to prevent disease. Patients who are already sick can be taught how to help the body heal itself. The school also offers three postgraduate courses on alternative medicines, including acupuncture, homeopathy, and natural medicine.

Illness Treated

All chronic degenerative diseases, such as cancer, arthritis, lupus, AIDS, diabetes, migraine, multiple sclerosis, allergies, conditions related to silicone breast implants, and chronic renal failure.

Treatment Offered

Approximately 216 different alternative therapies, including DMSO, chelation therapy with EDTA, shark cartilage, homeopathy, acupuncture, moxibustion, laser acupuncture, biofeedback, trace minerals treatment, amino acids, electromagnetism, electrolypolisis, massage, cocarboxilase, enzymes, nutrition therapy, megadoses of vitamins, colon therapy, live cell therapy, electroacupuncture according to Voll, neural therapy, ear medicine according to Nogier, Vega method, iridology, herbs, and homotoxicology. No single method is a cure-all, so different treatments are combined according to the needs of the patient. Orthodox medicine can also be used, but in small doses.

Related Readings

Enzimoterapia by Dr. Karl Ransberger and Dr. Hector Solorzano.

Length of Treatment/Stay

The more chronic the disease, the longer the stay. The longest stay is three weeks. Then the patient follows the program at home and can return if he or she wishes.

Costs

Costs not submitted for publication, but the means of the patient are considered.

Method of Payment

Checks or cash is accepted.

Revici Life Science Center

200 West 57th Street
Suite 1205
New York, New York 10019
United States

(212) 246-5122
Fax: (212) 246-1535

Contact Person

Elena Avram.

Primary Personnel

Kenneth Korms, M.D.; Emanuel Revici, M.D., available for consultations with physicians.

Directions

Located in midtown Manhattan, easily accessible by car and public transportation.

Background

Dr. Revici's treatments have been in evolution since the mid-1920s. His therapy is an outgrowth of his studies on lipids and their role in physiopathology. The agents are derived from natural sources or are synthesized to act like natural substances in the body. They are either lipidic or lipid-based and may incorporate various elements or metals (which are nontoxic in this form). The basic aim is to correct or control disorders in the body's defense systems. The Revici Life Science Center is outpatient only. There is no X-ray or CAT scan equipment on the premises, but those procedures are prescribed. Blood chemistries are also prescribed, although the actual analysis is done by outside labs. Urine samples and some blood samples are analyzed at the center.

Illness Treated

Dr. Revici has had some success with every type of cancer, even at late stages. The most spectacular cases appear to be long-term remissions in brain, lung, pancreatic, and metastasized breast carcinomas. The center also treats virtually all degenerative diseases, as well as AIDS.

Treatment Offered

Nontoxic chemotherapy, developed by Dr. Revici through original research over a period spanning nearly seven decades. The treatment is administered either orally, through drops in capsules, or by injection. The treatment is individually guided. The response seems to be individual.

Related Readings

Research in Physiopathology as Basis of Guided Chemotherapy With Special Application to Cancer by Emanuel Revici, M.D. Princeton, New Jersey: Van Nostrand Company Inc., 1961.

Emanuel Revici, M.D.: A Review of His Scientific Work by Dwight L. McKee, M.D., editor. Institute of Applied Biology, 1985.

Individuals interested in obtaining other publications by or about Dr. Revici should write to the center.

Length of Treatment/Stay

Variable, depending on stage of illness. The frequency of visits often is irregular. Most of the time, the patient, following instructions and keeping in touch by phone with the attending physician, administers the treatment at home.

Costs

First consultation, with treatment: $550. Repeat visits: $150. Autovaccination: $50.

Method of Payment

Cash and personal checks are accepted, except at the first consultation, where only cash or certified checks are accepted. Insurance companies have been honoring reimbursement requests on the whole. No assignments are accepted. Medication is free.

Vladimir Rizov, M.D.

8235 Shoal Creek Boulevard
Austin, Texas 78757
United States

(512) 451-8149

Primary Personnel

Vladimir Rizov, M.D.

Illness Treated

Cancer; best responder is prostate cancer. Dr. Rizov also treats cardiovascular problems, arthritis, allergies, chronic fatigue, fungal infections, and obesity, and he offers an anti-aging program.

Treatment Offered

Laetrile, orally and intravenously, with vitamin C, B complex, and DMSO; EDTA; enzymes; nutritional evaluation and correction; detoxification; chelation; oxygen therapy; and homeopathy.

Related Readings

Cancer and Vitamin C by Ewan Cameron and Linus Pauling. Linus Pauling Institute of Science and Medicine, 1979.

Bypassing Bypass by Elmer Cranton, M.D.

Length of Treatment/Stay

For cancer, six weeks. For other problems, variable length.

Costs

Introductory appointment: free. Six weeks of treatment: $7,000.

Method of Payment

Personal checks are accepted. Although the office will help the patient fill out insurance forms, it's up to the patient to collect reimbursement. Patients pay daily. Those who pay in advance for the full treatment will receive a 10 percent discount (nonrefundable).

Rosabell Medical Group

12732 W. Washington Boulevard, #D
Culver City, California 90066
United States

(310) 577-9338
Fax: (310) 822-0045

Contact Person

Huy Hoang, M.D.

Primary Personnel

Hans Gruenn, M.D.; Renee Garden.

Background

Doctors Hoang and Gruenn treat holistically and focus on preventive medicine.

Illness Treated

Treated illnesses include cancer, AIDS, CFIDS, gastrointestinal disturbances, candida, myalgia, and mercury toxicity.

Treatment Offered

Treatments include vitamin and mineral infusion therapy, intramuscular injections, nutritional counseling, and immune enhancement.

Length of Treatment/Stay

Varies, depending on the treatment.

Costs

Varies, depending on the treatment.

Method of Payment

Checks, cash, MasterCard, Visa, and Discover are accepted. Some insurance is accepted, including MetLife and Wellness Insurance.

Robert Rowen, M.D.

Omni Medical Center
615 E. 82nd Avenue, #300
Anchorage, Alaska 99518
United States

(907) 344-7775
Fax: (907) 522-3114

Contact Person

Bethany Buchanan, R.N., or Judy Cox, office manager.

Primary Personnel

Robert Rowen, M.D.; Joan Priestly, M.D.; William Stanley, R.D.; Ramon Gonzalez, L.A.C.

Illness Treated

Chronic pain, cancer, immune dysfunction, allergies, and cardiovascular diseases.

Treatment Offered

Chelation therapy, bio-oxidative therapy, nutrition, herbs, acupuncture, allergy elimination, detoxification, laetrile, 714X supervision, and others.

Length of Treatment/Stay

Three to four weeks.

Costs

Dependent upon treatment provided.

Method of Payment

Cash only is accepted.

The Ruscombe Mansion Community Health Center

4801 Yellowwood Avenue
Baltimore, Maryland 21209
United States

(410) 367-7300
Fax: (410) 356-6216

Contact Person

Zoh M. Hieronimus, founder and executive director.

Primary Personnel

Peter Hinderberger, M.D., Ph.D., medical director; Kathleen Galloway, R.N., director of acupuncture.

Directions

I-83 to Exit 9 Cold Spring Lane West. Right at light on Tamarind, follow winding road to Yellowwood. Turn left on Yellowwood, look for Ruscombe sign in parking lot on right.

Background

Founded in 1984 by Zoh Meyerhoff Hieronimus, the center provides a central location for practitioners of all types of holistic healing to operate their private practices. The center's goal is to support the natural healing process within the individual, emphasizing the use of nontoxic and noninvasive procedures. When working with a client, the practitioners at Ruscombe consider all aspects of the person—the physical, emotional, mental, and spiritual—for the achievement and maintenance of optimal health.

Illness Treated

Any and all illnesses are treated, including all kinds of cancer.

Treatment Offered

Treatments offered include homeopathy, anthroposophy, acupuncture, massage, counseling, Reiki, Trager, zero balancing, craniosacral therapy, and many others.

Length of Treatment/Stay

Length of treatment varies widely. This is an outpatient facility only.

Costs

Fees vary, depending on the treatment. For example, acupuncture is $50 per visit. Homeopathic consultation is $110 for the initial exam, and $35 for follow-up visits.

Method of Payment

Cash and checks are accepted. Insurance is accepted for some services. Payment is expected at the time of your visit.

The Rushing Clinic, P.A.

P.O. Box 57738
Webster, Texas 77598-7768
United States

(713) 286-2195
Fax: (713) 286-2197

Contact Person

Stephen O. Rushing, M.D.

Primary Personnel

Stephen O. Rushing, M.D.

Background

Dr. Rushing has been working actively with pain patients for three years.

Illness Treated

Cancer pain.

Treatment Offered

Pain management and treatment for cancer and other patients.

Length of Treatment/Stay

As needed.

Costs

Individual, $120 per hour.

Method of Payment

Cash, checks, Visa, and MasterCard are accepted. The clinic does not accept insurance assignments.

St. Joseph Medical Center

61 Avenue Rosas
Matamoros, Tamps
Mexico

011-52-88-161250
011-52-88-125344

Contact Person

Charles L. Rogers, M.D.

Primary Personnel

Charles L. Rogers, M.D., M.D.H., Chinese medicine practitioner.

Directions

Patients are transported daily from Brownsville, Texas.

Background

Since 1977, Dr. Rogers has done research to locate, use, and develop anything that will affect cancer in any form. He is a Doctor of Homeopathy (M.D.H.) as well as an M.D., and is also a practitioner and teacher of Chinese natural medicine. He draws on all of these approaches when treating his patients.

Illness Treated

Cancer and degenerative diseases.

Treatment Offered

Natural therapies to help prevent the diseased cells from spreading, followed by cancer-killing medications. At the same time, normal cells are given immune boosters to re-establish their normal reproductive capabilities, regenerating and strengthening the immune system. The treatments are based on a series of injections and infusions given daily, plus oral medications.

Related Readings

Information about past patients will be provided on request.

Length of Treatment/Stay

Varies with each patient. Typical stay is three to five weeks.

Costs

Sliding scale.

Method of Payment

Cash, checks, Visa, and MasterCard are accepted. Insurance is accepted; coverage depends on individual company.

Michael B. Schachter, M.D., P.C., and Associates

Two Executive Boulevard
Suite 202
Suffern, New York 10901
United States

(914) 368-4700
Fax: (914) 368-4727

Contact Person

Ask for new-patient educators.

Primary Personnel

Michael Schachter, M.D.; Philip Cohen, M.D.; A. Chu-Fong, M.D., oncologist; Bruce Oran, D.O.; Monica Furlong, M.D.; Sally Minniefield, certified physician's assistant; John J. Reynolds, certified physician's assistant; Shirley Ostro Gilad, R.N., F.N.P., and classical homeopath; Barbara Spreitzer, R.N., F.N.P.; Robert Connolly, licensed acupuncturist; Dolores Tritico, R.N., head nurse; Rommel Guerrero, laboratory director.

Directions

From points North: Take the New York State Thruway south (87 South-287 East) to Exit 14B Airmont Road. Turn left at the end of the exit ramp. Proceed to second traffic light and make left onto Executive Boulevard. The office is at the end on the right. From points South: Take the Thruway West (87 North-287 West) to Exit 14B Airmont Road. Turn right at the end of the exit ramp. At the next light, make a left onto Executive Boulevard. The office is at the end on the right. From New York City: Cross the George Washington Bridge on the upper level. Take the Palisades Parkway North to Exit 9 West, the New York State Thruway North. Follow directions as in "from points South." From New Jersey: Take the Garden State Parkway North to the N.Y. State Thruway toward "Albany-Suffern." Follow signs for Exits 14B-61 (87 North-287 West). Three miles past toll, take Exit 14B Airmont Road. Follow directions as in "from points South." Or: Take 287 North to signs to New York State Thruway. Bear right on 287. Exit onto 287 East-87 South toward Tappan Zee Bridge and New York City. Take Exit 14B Airmont Road, Suffern (Montebello). Follow directions as in "from points North." From Westchester and points East: Take the Thruway North across the Tappan Zee Bridge. Proceed on Thruway to Exit 14B Airmont Road. Follow directions as in "from points South."

Background

Dr. Schachter's practice, started in 1974, is based on a pragmatic philosophy combining the best of traditional medicine with alternative or holistic medicine. A variety of alternative treatments are integrated. The emphasis is on education, lifestyle changes, and the patient's taking responsibility for his or her treatment program by managing it on a partnership basis with his or her health care provider. This is an outpatient facility only, but in case of emergency, patients can be referred locally for inpatient care. Patients who are on programs with physicians outside the United States (such as Dr. Nieper and the various Mexican clinics) can receive support from Dr. Schachter and his associates.

Illness Treated

Cancer; the best responders are breast, lung, colon, lymphoma, and Hodgkin's disease. The center also treats AIDS, cardiovascular disorders, arthritis, allergies, candida-related complex, chronic fatigue syndrome, immune dysfunction, glandular disturbances, psychiatric disorders, neurological conditions, childhood disorders, gastro-intestinal disorders, gynecological disorders, musculoskeletal disorders, and patients who simply want a preventive health care program.

Treatment Offered

First, a complete medical history is taken; then there is a complete physical examination, followed by laboratory studies, which include routine blood and urine tests, special cancer markers, nutrient status assessment, an immune profile, and, when indicated, allergy testing. Nutritional and metabolic therapies are then used. Available therapies include orthomolecular medicine and psychiatry, psychotherapy, clinical ecology, preventive medicine, education, detoxification procedures, diet, nutritional supplements, exercise, stress management, and EDTA and DMPS chelation therapy. Emphasis is on injectable programs: intravenous vitamin C containing selected minerals and glutathione, amygdalin, DMSO, and intravenous hydrogen peroxide. Individual oral supplements may include vitamins, minerals, enzymes, amygdalin, shark cartilage, bovine tracheal cartilage, coenzyme Q_{10}, and concentrated herb extracts. Hydrazine sulfate is recommended for some cancer patients. Additional therapies include classical homeopathy, complex homeopathy, acupuncture, biomagnetic field therapy, therapeutic massage, saunas, bowel cleansing, and coffee enemas. Most supplements and other therapeutic devices can be purchased at the facility. Side effects are generally minimal. Work is also done with patients who are on chemotherapy under the care of other physicians.

Related Readings

Unconventional Cancer Treatments. U.S. Congress Office of Technology Assessment, September 1990.

Love, Medicine, and Miracles by Bernie Siegel, M.D. Harper & Row, 1986.

Cancer and Its Nutritional Therapies by Dr. Richard Passwater. Keats Publishing (revised edition), 1983.

International Protocols for Individualized, Integrated Metabolic Programs in Cancer Management by Robert W. Bradford, Michael Culbert, and Henry W. Allen. Robert W. Bradford Foundation, 1981.

The Cancer Industry: Unraveling the Politics by Ralph W. Moss. Paragon House, 1989. *Oxygen Therapies* by Ed McCabe. Energy Publications, 1988.

Biomagnetic Handbook by William H. Philpott, M.D., and Sharon Taplin. EnviroTech Products, 1990.

The Cancer Survivors by Judith Glassman. Dial Press, 1983.

The Metabolic Management of Cancer by Robert W. Bradford and Michael Culbert. Robert W. Bradford Foundation, 1979.

Making the Right Choice: Treatment Options in Cancer Surgery by Richard A. Evans, M.D. Avery Publishing Group, Inc., 1995.

The Complete Guide to Alternative Cancer Therapies: What You Need to Know to Make an Informed Choice by Ron Falcone. Carroll Publishing Group, 1994.

Save Yourself from Breast Cancer by Robert M. Kradjian, M.D. Berkley Books, 1994.

Cancer Therapy: The Independent Consumer's Guide to Non-Toxic Treatment and Prevention by Ralph W. Moss, Ph.D. Equinox Press, 1992.

Questioning Chemotherapy by Ralph W. Moss, Ph.D. Equinox Press, 1995.

Beating Cancer with Nutrition by Patrick Quillin, Ph.D., R.D. The Nutrition Times Press, Inc., 1994.

Dressed to Kill by Sydney Ross Singer. Avery Publishing Group, Inc., 1995.

Options: The Alternative Cancer Therapy Book by Richard Walters. Avery Publishing Group, Inc., 1993.

Length of Treatment/Stay

Two to three weeks for out-of-towners; locals (people from New York, New Jersey, or Connecticut) are seen regularly and followed up indefinitely.

Costs

Three weeks (without room and board): $1,500 to $3,000 for workup, counseling, and injectables program. Oral supplements: $100 to $1,000 per month; more occasionally.

Method of Payment

Cash, checks, money orders, and credit cards are accepted. The staff will help patients get third-party reimbursements but will not bill third-party insurers directly.

Schafer's Health Centre Ltd.

Box 251
Unity, Saskatchewan S0K 4L0
Canada

(306) 228-2512
Fax: (306) 228-4433

Primary Personnel

Dr. Sir Leo J. Schafer, M.H., R.H.C., L.C.S.P.

Directions

Corner of Highway 14 and Highway 21.

Background

After a prolonged illness, Schafer began studying the natural way of healing. He has read many books and attended many seminars and classes regarding reflexology, massage, iridology, herbology, magnetic therapy, color therapy, music and sound therapy, and radionics analysis. He received an honorary doctor's degree in homeopathy in 1984, and in 1985 he received his doctor's of medicine in holistic healing. On January 5, 1987, he became the seventeenth recipient of the Dag Hammarskjold award, and on August 30 that same year he was received into the order of the Royal Knights of Justice.

Illness Treated

Cancer and other diseases, including AIDS.

Treatment Offered

Herbology, color therapy, magnet therapy, music and sound therapy, diet, and nutrition. Dr. Schafer has over 220 of his own herbal formulas. Treatments may involve use of the Rife functional generator, which he makes and sells. He has been using these therapies for twenty years. There are few, if any, possible side effects.

Length of Treatment/Stay

One hour. This is an outpatient facility.

Costs

Consultation: $45 (plus tax). Program: $50 to $400 (plus tax).

Method of Payment

Cash, certified checks, and Visa are accepted.

Ron Schmid, N.D.

246 Federal Road, Suite 33A
Brookfield, Connecticut 06804
United States

(203) 740-1549

133 Reef Road
Fairfield, Connecticut 06830
United States

(203) 255-8195

Contact Person

Ellen Triplett.

Primary Personnel

Ronald F. Schmid, N.D., naturopathic physician; Ellen Triplett, clinical laboratory scientist (C.L.S.).

Directions

To Brookfield: Route 84 to Exit 7 (Route 7 North). Take first exit (Federal Road), go left at light, then make second right at Federal Road. Proceed north to #246, the "Brookfield Common" building.

Background

Dr. Schmid has specialized in nutritional medicine for over fifteen years. Each new patient is evaluated through a detailed medical and nutritional history and laboratory tests. A highly individualized and detailed program is worked out with each patient. Dr. Schmid has studied and integrated the work of Max Gerson, Weston Price, and other pioneer researchers in natural therapies for cancer and other chronic diseases.

Illness Treated

All types of cancer; autoimmune problems such as lupus and rheumatoid arthritis; osteoarthritis; colitis and irritable bowel syndrome; ulcers, gastritis; skin diseases, such as eczema and psoriasis; allergies; and virtually all chronic diseases.

Treatment Offered

Treatment is primarily dietary, complemented by supplements specific to the individual and the medical problem. Diet is highly individualized but natural foods-based, emphasizing raw greens and vegetables, certain fish and other high-quality protein, some fresh fruit, and often specific juices. Supplements include the best that recent research indicates.

Related Readings

Native Nutrition: Eating According to Ancestral Wisdom by Ronald Schmid, N.D.

Length of Treatment/Stay

One to three years of intensive diet and supplements; lifelong natural foods diet thereafter.

Costs

First visit, one-and-a-half hours, $225; subsequent visits, one hour, $150. Lab work, typically $125 to $500. Supplements recommended vary according to means of patient, can range from about $125 a month to as much as $1,500 to $2,000, depending on the case.

Method of Payment

Cash, checks, MasterCard, and Visa are accepted. Most insurance plans reimburse for the doctor's services, but the office requires payment from the patient at the time of the visit.

Ahmad Shamim, M.D.

200 Fort Meade Road
Laurel, Maryland 20707
United States

(301) 776-3700 *(D.C. area)*
(410) 792-0333 *(Baltimore, MD area)*

Contact Person

Elizabeth.

Primary Personnel

Ahmad Shamim, M.D.

Directions

From Washington, D.C., take Baltimore-Washington Parkway north. Take exit for Route 197. Turn left on Route 197 toward Laurel. Drive three miles to the Steward Towers high-rise apartment building, 200 Ft. Meade Road., at the intersection of 197 and 198.

Background

Dr. Shamim was trained as a general surgeon. Since 1976, he has gradually changed his practice to nutrition-based, holistic, preventive medicine. He primarily treats chronic degenerative diseases, including cancer, using nontoxic, natural, nutritional, and herbal remedies. On the first visit, the patient is interviewed extensively by the doctor, and then has a physical exam. The nurse then explains the regimen in detail.

Illness Treated

Chronic degenerative diseases, including cancer, heart disease, hypertension, arthritis, diabetes, asthma, allergies, digestive disorders, chronic fatigue, depression, yeast-related illnesses, and multiple sclerosis.

Treatment Offered

Emphasis is on cleansing and detoxifying the body, then stimulating and enhancing the immune system. All natural herbal products and a special intestinal cleansing program are outlined. A strict diet and fresh organic vegetable juices are emphasized. Enzymes, minerals, and vitamins of specific kinds and dosages; glandular products; fatty acids; herbal medications; injections of vitamins and minerals, including intravenous vitamin C in large doses; and anti-yeast medications are used.

Related Readings

Cancer and Vitamin C by Ewan Cameron and Linus Pauling.
Dr. Max Gerson's book on cancer therapy.

Length of Treatment/Stay

Varies, depending on the illness and the patient's condition.

Costs

Very reasonable charges for office visits and injections. Call for details.

Method of Payment

Cash and checks are accepted. Insurance is not accepted, but forms are completed and given to the patient.

Shealy Institute for Comprehensive Health Care

1328 East Evergreen
Springfield, Missouri 65803
United States

(417) 865-5940
Fax: (417) 865-6111

Contact Person

C. Norman Shealy, M.D., Ph.D.

Primary Personnel

C. Norman Shealy, M.D., Ph.D.; Roger K. Cady, M.D.; Kenneth L. Everett, R.N.; Kathleen Farmer, Psy.D.; Diane Veehoff, R.N., M.S.W.

Directions

South of Highway I-44, in north Springfield, Missouri.

Background

The institute began in 1971 as the first comprehensive pain clinic in the country. It has expanded to include comprehensive health care of all kinds. It has a multidisciplinary team with a staff of twenty-eight highly dedicated, holistically oriented individuals. Their philosophy is to apply all conceivable, safe approaches. Traditional approaches are used when appropriate. The institute provides treatment programs up to eight hours per day for up to twenty patients.

Illness Treated

All illnesses excluding acute psychosis. Cancer is among the disorders treated. Contact the center to find out the location of its AIDS treatment center.

Treatment Offered

Biogenics, individual counseling, massage, nutritional counseling, biofeedback training, acupuncture, consultations, drug detoxification, electrosleep therapy, facet rhizotomy, nerve blocks, Sarapin injections, smoking control, transcutaneous electrical nerve stimulation, and musical vibration for deep relaxation.

Length of Treatment/Stay

Fifteen days for most chronic problems; sometimes shorter, and occasionally longer.

Related Readings

Creation of Health by C. Norman Shealy, M.D., Ph.D., and Caroline Myss, M.A.
90 Days to Self-Help by C. Norman Shealy, M.D. Second edition, 1987.
The Pain Game by C. Norman Shealy, M.D. Element Publishing, 1976.
Miracles Do Happen by C. Norman Shealy, M.D. Element Publishing.

Costs

Approximately $4,000 for two weeks of therapy.

Method of Payment

Cash, checks, money orders, and credit cards are accepted. The institute will assist patients in filing insurance, but does not take insurance assignments.

Sierra Clinic Inc.

30003 Gobernador Logo, Suite 202
Tijuana, B.C.
Mexico

011-52-66-864672

Appointments, Reservations, or Details:
P.O. Box 3177
Walnut Creek, California 94598
United States

(510) 935-0162
(619) 422-6261

Contact Person

Mrs. Rory Dominguez. Free brochure sent on request.

Primary Personnel

G.J. Palafox, M.D.

Directions

Directions are given at the All Seasons Inn, 699 "E" St. #118, Chula Vista, California, United States.

Background

The Sierra Clinic is operated by Dr. Palafox, who has been practicing in Tijuana for more than thirty-three years. Dr. Palafox was also managing director of a Catholic nuns' hospital in Tijuana for more than seventeen years. He has treated hundreds of terminal and nonterminal cancer patients. The clinic admits only ambulatory patients into its three-week treatment. These treatments are nontoxic and are said to have no side effects or after-effects. After treatment, the patients are given instructions to help them maintain their immune systems at optimum levels. After a complete medical history has been taken and a medical exam has been completed, the patients start treatment the following day, except on Sundays. During treatment, many patients stay in Chula Vista at the All Seasons Inn, which provides transportation to the clinic and back. Departure for the clinic is usually at 9:30 a.m., and the patient is back at the inn at about 11 p.m.

Illness Treated

Cancer, arthritis, and Down's syndrome.

Treatment Offered

A homeopathic detoxification program, chelation, amino acid supplementation (L-arginine), and daily injections of vitamins and minerals. For Down's syndrome patients, the clinic uses the protocol developed by Dr. Nicolas Weinstien of Santiago, Chile, and Dr. Henry Turkel, a series of amino acid injections and oral formulas.

Length of Treatment/Stay

Eighteen days, or eighteen injections.

Costs

Cancer treatment: $6,400, which includes medication and six months of home maintenance. Down's syndrome treatment: $4,200, including a year of injections and oral medication.

Method of Payment

Cashier's checks, approved personal checks, money orders, and credit cards are accepted.

Charles Simone, M.D.

Simone Protective Cancer Center
123 Franklin Corner Road
Lawrenceville, New Jersey 08648
United States

(609) 896-2646

Contact Person

Charles B. Simone, M.D.

Directions

Exit 8A off Interstate 95.

Background

Medical oncologist (National Cancer Institute), tumor immunologist, radiation oncologist.

Illness Treated

All cancers, precancers, and cardiovascular disease.

Treatment Offered

Adjunctive therapies, including hormonal treatments.

Related Readings

Cancer and Nutrition by Charles B. Simone, M.D. Avery Publishing Group, 1992
Breast Health by Charles B. Simone, M.D. Avery Publishing Group, 1995

Length of Treatment/Stay

Varies, depending on condition.

Costs

Varies, depending on condition.

Method of Payment

Medical insurance covers physician and procedure costs.

Suzanne Skinner, Ph.D.

2204 Torrance Boulevard, Suite 101
Torrance, California 90501
United States

(310) 518-4555

Contact Person

Dr. Suzanne M. Skinner, Ph.D., R.N.C., N.D., D.Sc., C.H.

Primary Personnel

Pat, Sally, Sharon, Theresa, and Fasoli (counseling and support).

Illness Treated

All illnesses are treated. The therapies get the body in balance after detoxification, enabling the body to heal itself.

Treatment Offered

Contact Reflex Analysis, which reveals deficiencies based on the strength of the patient's reflexes, is used to determine the root cause of a health problem. Once this cause is known, structural and/or nutritional support is given to help the body heal itself. Treatments include colonics, homeopathy, herbs, whole foods, supplements, and lymphatic work.

Length of Treatment

Varies.

Costs

Initial visit: $175; $45 thereafter. Supplements are extra.

Method of Payment

Cash, Visa, MasterCard, Discover, and American Express are accepted.

Georg F. Springer, M.D.

Heather M. Bligh Cancer Research Laboratories
UHS/Chicago Medical School
3333 Green Bay Road
North Chicago, Illinois 60064
United States

(708) 578-3435
(708) 578-3432

Contact Person

Shelia Carlstedt.

Primary Personnel

Georg F. Springer, M.D., D.Sc.hc; Parimal R. Desai, Ph.D; Baole Wang, M.D.;
Max Goldschmidt, M.D.

Illness Treated

Breast cancer.

Treatment Offered

Immunological.

Costs

Costs depend on the financial status of the patient. Services may be free.

Stella Maris Clinic

P.O. Box 435123
San Ysidro, California 92143
United States

(800) 662-1319
011-52-66-343444

Contact Person

Gilberto Alvarez, M.D.

Primary Personnel

Complete medical staff including all specialties, providing twenty-four-hour service on
an inpatient basis.

Directions

The clinic is located only three minutes from the international border in New Zona Rio in Tijuana, at Edmundo O'Gorman 1571, Tijuana, B.C., Mexico, one block after Cuahtecmoc Monument. Transportation is provided to and from the San Diego Airport.

Background

The Stella Maris Clinic offers help for the cancer patient as well as those with other degenerative diseases, through natural methods and nutritional support. Its clinical experience of more than seventeen years has shown satisfactory results in the treatment and prevention of malignant and non-malignant degenerative diseases, as well as immunological disorders.

Illness Treated

Mostly neoplastic conditions, with best results in breast, prostate, and lung cancer; lymphomas; and brain tumors.

Treatment Offered

Alternative methods, including detoxification, enzyme therapy, and amygdalin (B_{17}), as well as building up the immune system.

Related Readings

Based on Dr. Harold Manner's protocols.

Length of Treatment/Stay

Twenty-one days.

Costs

$3,300 per week, including treatments, room and board, and diagnostic studies such as CAT scans, MRI, X-rays, and blood work.

Method of Payment

Cashier's checks are accepted.

Valley Cancer Institute

12099 West Washington Boulevard
Suite 304
Los Angeles, California 90066-0549
United States

(310) 398-0013
Fax: (310) 398-4470

Contact Person

Tressia Keen, B.S.N., M.N., patient information coordinator.

Primary Personnel

James Bicher, M.D., medical director.

Directions

Take the 405 freeway south to the Culver/Braddock exit or north to the Washington Boulevard exit.

Background

Founded in 1985, the Valley Cancer Institute is the largest hyperthermic oncology (the use of locally applied heat to destroy tumors) research and patient treatment center in the country. The institute contains the most advanced hyperthermic technology equipment, including microwave and ultrasound, and a linear accelerator and simulator. It also has research laboratories and both inpatient and outpatient treatment facilities.

Illness Treated

Cancer, including adenocarcinoma, carcinoma, melanoma, thymoma, squamous cell carcinoma, mesothelioma, sarcoma, lymphoma, basal cell cancer, skin cancer, Kaposi's sarcoma (including AIDS-related), and BPH (benign prostate hyperplasia). Effective treatable sites include the brain, bones, throat, thyroid, lungs, breast, liver, pancreas, colon, ovaries, uterus, prostate, and others.

Treatment Offered

Hyperthermia is basically nontoxic, reduces pain, and lessens the side effects of standard treatments. The institute also provides nutritional information and educational support.

Related Readings

Dr. Bicher has written eight books and more than 230 articles in professional medical and engineering journals. Call for exact titles.

Length of Treatment/Stay

Varies from patient to patient, but a typical treatment lasts eight weeks, five days per week, one to two hours per day.

Costs

Costs, not submitted for publication, will vary depending on the extent of the cancer and the number of fields of treatment required.

Method of Payment

Most private insurance pays; the treatment is approved for reimbursement through Medicare. Call for further details.

Vital-Life Institute

P.O. Box 294
Encinitas, California 92024
United States

(619) 943-8485
Fax: (619) 436-9642

Contact Person

Patty Harper.

Primary Personnel

Steven R. Schechter, N.D., Ph.D.

Directions

The institute is near highway I-5, along the ocean, between La Costa Avenue and Leucadia Boulevard, thirty minutes north of San Diego Airport, and one hour south of Anaheim.

Background

Dr. Schechter is the author of a book on natural remedies that strengthen the immune system; detoxify the body from chemical pollutants, radiation, X-rays, drugs, and alcohol; generate maximum vitality and health; and prevent or treat disease—including cancer. Dr. Schechter has been the featured speaker at health industry trade conventions and consumer health expos. He was director of clinical nutrition and medical herbology at a large medical detoxification clinic. Health consultations are offered in person, on an outpatient basis, or over the telephone. All information is based on extensive clinical experience and upon thousands of primary scientific research studies documenting the safety and effectiveness of specific natural remedies.

Illness Treated

Cancers, including breast, lung, liver, lymph, pancreas, colon, cervix, uterus, and prostate; tumors, including brain tumors; AIDS and CFIDS; Epstein-Barr virus; yeast infection; liver-related disorders; environmental injury; and other disorders related to immune deficiency.

Treatment Offered

Therapeutic foods, herbs, vitamin and mineral supplements, amino acids, glandular extracts, enzymes, periodic short fasts, exercise programs, positive visualizations, and other natural remedies.

Related Readings

Fighting Radiation & Chemical Pollutants With Foods, Herbs, & Vitamins: Documented Natural Remedies That Boost Your Immunity & Detoxify by Steven R. Schechter, N.D.

Length of Treatment/Stay

Most treatments are on an outpatient basis or over the telephone. People may call for a telephone consultation or come to Vital-Life and stay at a nearby hotel or motel. The center is open from 11 a.m. to 3 p.m.

Costs

Consultation fee: $95 per hour.

Method of Payment

Checks, cash, money orders, Visa, and MasterCard are accepted. Some insurance companies will reimburse the client.

Waisbren Clinic

2315 North Lake Drive
Suite 815
Milwaukee, Wisconsin 53211
United States

(414) 272-1929

Contact Person

Robyn.

Primary Personnel

Burton A. Waisbren Sr., M.D.

Directions

From Chicago, take Highway 43 north to Milwaukee. Go east on North Avenue until you get to Seton Tower at St. Mary's Hospital.

Background

The Waisbren Clinic believes that surgery, radiation, chemotherapy, immunotherapy, and nutrition are all important in cancer treatment. The clinic's main focus, however, is immunotherapy, which is meant to increase the efficiency of the immune system to help the body fight cancer.

Illness Treated

Carcinoma, lymphoma, multiple sclerosis, and chronic fatigue syndrome.

Treatment Offered

BCG, Coley's vaccine, lymphoblastoid lymphocytes, autogenous vaccine, transfer factor, Interleukin2, and Interferon.

Length of Treatment/Stay

Once every other week for eight weeks, then monthly with self-administered Interleukin2, Interferon, and bacterial vaccines.

Costs

Approximately $400 to $600 per visit.

Method of Payment

Cash or credit cards are accepted. The clinic submits insurance, but few companies will reimburse the patient.

Warren's Clinic

7171 Airline Highway, Suite 1
Baton Rouge, Louisiana 70805
United States

(504) 355-3741

Contact Person

Nicole or Dr. Warren.

Primary Personnel

J.D. Warren, D.C., N.D. Holistic Health Doctor degree.

Directions

Five blocks off Airline Highway.

Background

Dr. Warren has been at this facility for ten years and has been practicing his therapy for fifteen years. He believes in treating the person, not the disease.

Illness Treated

Cancer and other degenerative diseases, including AIDS, early Alzheimer's disease, heart and circulatory diseases, emphysema, allergies, prostate troubles, diabetes, osteoporosis, osteomyelitis, and others.

Treatment Offered

Nutritional—herbal, homeopathic, glandular, and others

Related Readings

Treating AIDS Nutritionally by Dr. Lawrence Bagly, M.D.

Length of Treatment/Stay

Depends on the body's response.

Costs

Very conservative.

Method of Payment

Cash, checks, Visa, MasterCard, and insurance are accepted. The patient pays what insurance does not.

Julian Whitaker, M.D.

4321 Birch Street, Suite 100
Newport Beach, California 92660
United States

(714) 851-1550
Fax: (714) 851-9970

Contact Person

Clinic communication director.

Primary Personnel

Allan E. Sosin, M.D.; J.W. Thompsen, M.D.

Directions

Near John Wayne Airport, Orange County, California.

Illness Treated

Heart disease, diabetes, arthritis, and hormone replacement.

Treatment Offered

Five-and-a-half week resident program.

Related Readings

Reversing Diabetes.
Reversing Heart Disease.
Guide to Natural Healing.
Is Heart Surgery Necessary?

Costs

$1,200.

Method of Payment

Visa, MasterCard, and Medicare are accepted.

Woodlands Medical Center, Inc.

5724 Clymer Road
Quakertown, Pennsylvania 18951
United States

(215) 536-1890

Contact Person

Harold E. Buttram, M.D.

Primary Personnel

Harold E. Buttram, M.D., family practice and environmental medicine; William Kracht, D.O., family practice, obstetrics, environmental medicine; Richard Piccola, administrative director, M.H.A.

Directions

Woodlands Medical Center is approximately thirty-five miles north of Philadelphia, near Quakertown. From Quakertown, take Highway 313 east. About three miles outside of Quakertown, you will come to a Wagon Wheel Tavern on the right. Take a black-topped road angling off to the left here. Go about half a mile to the next crossroad, which is Clymer Road, and turn left. Go another half a mile; Woodlands Medical Center is on the right.

Background

At the center, emphasis is placed on proper nutrition, avoidance of potentially toxic environmental chemicals, and personal responsibility in health care. Prescription medications are used when considered necessary, but the "natural" approaches are preferred and used in large measure.

Illness Treated

In children: routine health care, attention deficit hyperactive syndrome, autism, and allergies. In adults: chronic fatigue, immune dysfunction disorders, environmental illness (multiple chemical sensitivity), allergies, family practice, obstetrics and preconception care.

Treatment Offered

Chelation therapy, allergy neutralization therapy based on serial dilution titration technique, enzyme potentiated desensitization, preconception and obstetrics, nutritional counseling, and homeopathy.

Related Readings

It Is Only Natural by Gerald Poesnecker, D.O.

One Flesh by Gerald Poesnecker, D.O.

For Tomorrow's Children by Harold Buttram, M.D.

Our Toxic World: Who Is Looking After Our Kids? Harold Buttram, M.D. and Richard Piccola, M.H.A.

Length of Treatment/Stay

For major allergy problems, the usual length of therapy is one to three years. Chelation therapy is usually given in courses of twenty weekly treatments. Additional treatments may be needed depending on the condition being treated.

Costs

Generally, the center tries to keep costs as low as possible, so as to be affordable for the average family. The cost of a course of chelation is about $3,500. The initial cost for allergy treatment is $400 to $500, including the initial examination and testing. It averages $100 to $120 per month afterwards. Laboratory tests are extra, but are often covered by insurance. Enzyme potentiated desensitization is less expensive.

Method of Payment

Cash, checks, Visa, and MasterCard are accepted. The center also accepts Blue Cross and Blue Shield, and bills insurance for laboratory tests whenever possible.

Ray Wunderlich Jr., M.D.

666 6th Street South, Suite 206
St. Petersburg, Florida 33701
United States

(813) 822-3612

Illness Treated

Dementia, cancers, allergies, nutrient disorders, hyperactivity, attention deficit disorders, toxicities, cardiovascular diseases, and hypertension.

Treatment Offered

Chelation, supplements, and herbs.

Costs

Cost are open.

Method of Payment

Payment methods are open.

S. Yurkovsky, M.D.

309 Madison Street
Westbury, New York 11590
United States

(516) 333-2929

Primary Personnel

All services are provided by Dr. Yurkovsky personally.

Directions

Northern State Parkway, Exit 32 S.

Background

The doctor has worked for ten years in alternative medicine. He provides a strictly individualized approach based on bio-resonance testing and applied kinesiology, followed by homeopathic and Chinese herbals to detoxify and restore blocked energy pathways and circulation.

Illness Treated

All general medical problems, from cancer, chronic fatigue, and ecological illnesses to emotional-mental disorders and infertility.

Treatment Offered

Darkfield microscopy, homotoxicology, chelation therapy, homeopathy, intravenous ozone treatment, clinical nutrition, referrals for acupuncture and osteopathic treatments.

Related Readings

Guide to Alternative Therapies.

Length of Treatment/Stay

Strictly individualized, from a few weeks to months.

Costs

First visit: $385. Includes detailed history, physical exam, darkfield microscopy, and initial applied kinesiology assessment. Any tests, blood work, X-rays, etc. are kept to a minimum, if any, and referred out.

Victoria Zupa, N.D.

685 Post Road
Darien, Connecticut 06820
United States

(203) 656-4300
Fax: (203) 656-3050

Primary Personnel

Victoria Zupa, N.D.

Directions

From 95 going north get off at Exit 11. At the stop sign, make a left onto Route 1 North, which turns into Route 1 East and is also called Post Road. Follow this for an eighth of a mile. You will pass Darien Sports Shop, go under the railroad station, and pass the fire station on the right. Shortly after this, you will see a sign on the left that says Darien Chiropractic Center. Make a left into the driveway and park in the back; the entrance is in front. From 95 going south, get off at Exit 13. At the stop sign, make a left onto Route 1 West, which is also called Post Road. Follow this for a sixth of a mile. There are no signs. You will pass Darien Golf Center, Grant's Auto Body, and Four Seasons Farm Deli on the right. Shortly after this, you will see a sign on the right that says Darien Chiropractic Center. Make a right into the driveway, and park in the back; the entrance is in front.

Background

Dr. Victoria Zupa is a naturopathic physician trained as a specialist in alternative (natural) medicine at Bastyr University, a four-year, graduate-level naturopathic medical school. Dr. Zupa also has four years of pre-med and holds a B.A. in psychology. Although educated in the conventional medical sciences, and licensed by the State of Connecticut to practice naturopathic medicine, she is not an M.D. Dr. Zupa carries an N.D. (Doctor of Naturopathic Medicine).

Illness Treated

Cancer and immune system disorders.

Treatment Offered

Clinical nutrition, homeopathic medicine, botanical medicine, physical medicine, exercise therapy, counseling and stress management, and hydrotherapy. These treatments are tailored to the needs of the individual patient. As a naturopathic physician, Dr. Zupa will interface with all other branches of medical science.

Length of Treatment/Stay

Depends upon the condition.

Costs

Initial visit (one hour and fifteen minutes): $180. Office visits: $120/hour. Telephone consultation: $120/hour. These fees are approximate and will vary depending on the complexity of the case.

Method of Payment

Checks, cash, money orders, and Connecticut Blue Cross/Blue Shield are accepted. Payment is expected at the time of treatment. The office does not accept assignment from insurance companies.

TREATMENT CENTERS

Hospitals, Clinics, Physicians, Health Practitioners
Overseas (Germany, Hong Kong, Ireland, Israel, Japan,
New Zealand, Portugal, Spain, Switzerland, United Kingdom)

Hartmut Baltin, M.D.

Zellerhornstr. 3
83229 Aschau
Germany

011-08052-4176
Fax: 011-08052-905817

Primary Personnel

Hartmut Baltin, M.D.

Directions

Between Salzburg and Munich, three kilometers (about two miles) to the Autobahn A9 (Highway 1), located in a beautiful mountain village.

Background

Baltin takes a holistic approach to illness, including traditional German naturopathic medicine; Japanese and Chinese medicine; homeopathic and different kinds of osteopathic medicine, including ozone therapy; Carnivora; minerals; vitamins; and oxygen. Diagnostics are centered on focal problems, such as teeth.

Illness Treated

Cancer, multiple sclerosis, HIV, autoimmune diseases, and chronic pain.

Treatment Offered

For cancer treatment, surgery, diet, plant extracts, hyperthermia, ozone, vaccinations, minerals, vitamins, psychotherapy, and acupuncture are offered. Pain control is also offered.

Related Readings

Killing Pain Without Prescription.

Length of Treatment/Stay

Two to six weeks

Costs

Costs depend on illness and treatment.

Method of Payment

Cash, Visa, and MasterCard are accepted Dr. Baltin is a member of TRICARE Europe.

Bay of Plenty Environmental Health Clinic

157 Fraser Street
Tauranga
New Zealand

011-07-578-5899
Fax: 011-07-578-2362

Primary Personnel

Mike Godfrey, M.B.B.S.

Background

The clinic specializes in environmental and preventive medicine.

Illness Treated

Cancer, Alzheimer's disease, cardiovascular disorders, and other chronic diseases.

Treatment Offered

Nutritional and immunosupportive therapies for chronic diseases and cancer, using German and Scandinavian protocols. Mercury amalgam investigations, and safe detoxification with amalgam removal in a mercury-free dental clinic. Chelation therapy for cardiovascular disorders, Alzheimer's disease, and chemical detoxification. Acupuncture and homeopathy.

Costs

Overall costs are one-third of most European and North American clinics.

Bio Med Klinik
(Hospital for Applied Immunology and Biomedicine)

Tischberger Str. 5-8
D-76887 Bad Borgzabern
Germany

011-634-37050

Contact Person

E. Dieter Hager, M.D., Ph.D.

Primary Personnel

Mrs. Ulrike Modrzynski.

Background

The clinic has been open since 1989, and has 125 beds.

Illness Treated

Cancer and immunodeficiencies, such as chronic fatigue syndrome.

Treatment Offered

Conventional, complementary, and alternative therapy, including chemotherapy, hormone therapy, hyperthermia, fever therapy, active specific immunotherapy (ASI/tumor vaccination), nonspecific immunotherapy, thymus peptides, mistletoe, electrotherapy (galvanotherapy), and psychotherapy.

Related Readings

Biological Cancer Therapy.

Length of Treatment/Stay

Two to four weeks.

Costs

$350 to $500 U.S.*

Method of Payment

Cash and checks are accepted.

*Subject to the value of the U.S. dollar abroad.

Joseph Brenner, M.D.

46 Heh Iyar Street
Tel-Aviv
Israel

011-03-5467733
Fax: 011-03-5441296

Contact Person

Joseph Brenner, M.D.

Background

Dr. Brenner is the head of the conventional medical oncology unit in Tel-Aviv. He spent three years at Memorial Sloan Kettering Hospital in New York. In his private practice, he treats cancer patients with nutritional and psychological support, and different types of alternative methods.

Illness Treated

Mainly cancer.

Treatment Offered

Nutrition; megadoses of vitamins and minerals, including vitamin C; B_{17} (laetrile); iscador, shark cartilage, neytumorin, carcinomium compostium (HEEL); herbs; Chinese medicine; acupuncture; NSAIDs; and more.

Length of Treatment/Stay

Length depends on the specific program. One to three hours, one to two times a week.

Costs

$100 to $1,000 U.S.* a month, depending on the program.

Method of Payment

Cash, checks, and credit cards are accepted.

*Subject to the value of the U.S. dollar abroad.

The Bristol Cancer Help Centre

Clifton, Bristol BS8 4PG
England
United Kingdom

011-44-117-980-9500 (from the United States)
0117-980-9500 (from England)
0117-980-9527/28/29 (telephone counseling from England)

Contact Person

Receptionist for general inquiries; Helen Cooke, patient services manager; Graham Campbell, information services.

Primary Personnel

Dr. R.M. Daniel, B.Sc., M.B.B.Ch., centre director and medical director.

Directions

By train from London: Paddington Station to Bristol (Temple Meads) Station. By car from London: M4 westward, M32 into Bristol.

Background

Located in Bristol, one-and-a-half hours due west of London, the centre was originally opened in 1980 as an outpatient clinic. In 1983 it was relocated and expanded to an inpatient facility. The clinic is not suitable for people who are nonambulatory or in severe pain.

Illness Treated

Cancer, all types.

Treatment Offered

A holistic program of complementary therapies that stimulate the immune system and revitalize the natural self-healing process. The program can be safely used alongside orthodox medical treatment. The therapy is geared to the whole person: body, mind, and spirit. An organic natural diet supplemented by vitamins and minerals, herbal extracts, and Bach Flower Remedies greatly assists in the self-healing process. Relaxation, meditation, imagery, and visualization calm both body and mind. Individual counseling and spiritual healing harmonize emotions and spirit. Patients are helped to change their orientation and lifestyle. Nutritional advice, creative expression (through art therapy, movement, and sound), shiatsu, and massage also play a very important part in the program. The centre does not profess to offer a cure for cancer; its emphasis is on improving the quality of life.

Related Readings

Loving Medicine by Dr. Rosy Daniel.
Gentle Giants by Penny Brohn. London: Century Publishing.
The Bristol Programme by Penny Brohn.
Fighting Spirit edited by Heather Goodare. London: Scarlet Press.
Cancer and Nutrition—The Positive Scientific Evidence by Dr. Rosy Daniel and Dr. Sandra Goodman.
Healing Foods by Dr. Rosy Daniel. London: Thorsons Publishers
Healing Foods Cookbook by Jane Sen. London: Thorsons Publishers.

Length of Treatment/Stay

One day minimum. One week recommended

Costs

Introductory day: patient £50, supporter £25. Residential week: patient £475, supporter £225. Follow-up day: patient £75, supporter £25. These costs cover doctors' and therapists' consultations, therapy treatments, meals, etc. There are also Doctors' Phone-Ins, which are pre-booked and are free.

Method of Payment

Cash, checks, banker's drafts, Visa, and MasterCard are accepted.

The East Clinic

Thomas Street
Killaloe, County Clare
Ireland

011-353-61-376349
Fax: 011-353-61-376773

Contact Person

Paschal Carmody, M.B.

Primary Personnel

Paschal Carmody, M.B., B.Ch., D.C.H., D.Obs.

Directions

The clinic is located thirty miles from Shannon Airport, five miles off the main N7 Limerick/Dublin Road.

Background

The clinic was established twenty years ago, and has fifty-five beds.

Illness Treated

Cancer; cardiovascular disease; and musculoskeletal, dermatological, hematological, and neurological therapies.

Treatment Offered

Immune modulating treatments, including live cell treatment; ozone treatment; total-body hyperthermia with low-dose chemotherapy; local hyperthermia; chelation treatment; and nutritional supplement treatment.

Length of Treatment/Stay

From two to five weeks.

Costs

£1,500 per week. Live cell therapy is extra.

Method of Payment

Cash, checks, and Visa are accepted.

J. Buxalleu Font

Carrer d'Avall No. 44
08350 Arenys de Mar
Barcelona
Spain

011-93-792-0489

Contact Person

J. Buxalleu Font.

Directions

By car: Arrive at Arenys de Mar from Barcelona from the toll road (direction of Mataro). Keep going straight along Highway N-11 to Arenys de Mar. By Train: The railway begins at the airport of Barcelona (C-4 line), crosses Barcelona and runs along the coast. Arenys de Mar is about forty kilometers (twenty-four miles) from Barcelona, in the northeast direction.

Background

This is an outpatient clinic only. This therapy has been in use since 1965 without any side effects.

Illness Treated

Cancer only (solid tumors). Sometimes the localization is more important than the type of tumor; liver and brain cancers are difficult.

Treatment Offered

Self-vaccination. The patient's blood is extracted periodically, modified, and injected back into the patient with gamma globulin. In addition, treatment with a new personal construction molecule has recently begun. It increases immunity while being an antibiotic to malignant cells and nontoxic to normal cells.

Related Readings

A few articles have been published in Spanish journals. The center will provide upon request information regarding past patients.

Length of Treatment/Stay

The minimum length of stay is about three months. The recommended length is indefinite. In three months, with intensive treatment, the metabolic alteration of the organism is curbed. Extending this treatment over several years, the metabolic alteration may be rectified.

Costs

The cost depends on the patient's economic status. The cost of the vaccine together with the complementary treatment is about $600 U.S.* a month.

Method of Payment

Cash only is accepted. No insurance or credit cards are accepted.

---

*Subject to the value of the U.S. dollar abroad.

Health Center of Lisbon

Rua de Misericordia, #137-1
1200 Lisbon
Portugal

011-351-1-347-1117
Fax: 011-351-1-347-1111

Contact Person

Serge Jurasunas, N.D.

Primary Personnel

Two medical doctors, two naturopaths, one osteopath, one acupuncturist, and one nurse.

Background

The center was established fifteen years ago by Serge Jurasunas, a practitioner of naturopathic medicine, biology, nutrition, and iridology. His area of research today includes molecular biology, hematology, and cancer. He holds degrees in naturopathy, homeopathy, and biology. For over ten years, he has conducted research on oxycology and blood observation, including live blood analysis. These methods are used at the center, together with other types of holistic diagnosis.

Illness Treated

Cancer, especially of the breast, stomach, prostate, colon, pancreas, and brain. Also degenerative diseases such as multiple sclerosis, Parkinson's disease, and chronic fatigue syndrome.

Treatment Offered

Geoxy 132, chitin, Ukraine therapy, bamboo leaf extract, S.G.E., aloe vera injections, special magnetic mineral water, xian tian therapy, propermyl, L.E.M., tributyrrate, peptide, live cell therapy, D.M.S.O., hematoxilan, physiatrons, ophio therapy, nucleic acid, autolysat of human bacteria, enzymatic therapies adjuvant to the oxidative system, glutathione cysteine, S.O.D., and taurine injectable therapies. Detoxification is also important in the center'streatment.

Related Readings

Germanium, an Answer to Cancer by Serge Jurasunas.

Length of Treatment/Stay

Varies, depending on the type and stage of the disease.

Costs

Complete check-up: $150 U.S. (including all tests and diagnosis). The cost of the treatment varies between $500 to $1,000 U.S. per week. At-home treatment varies between $1,000 to $2,000 U.S. monthly. At present, the center does not accept any inpatients. It provides rooms near the health center for aproximately $60 U.S.* per day.

Method of Payment

Cash only is accepted.

*Subject to the value of the U.S. dollar abroad.

Holistic Keihoku Hospital

1-32-3 Sugamo
Toshimaku
Tokyo 170
Japan

011-03-3946-7271
Fax: 011-03-3917-9753

Contact Person

Tsuneo Kobayashi, M.D., director.

Background

The hospital offers a multidisciplinary treatment, artificial realization of spontaneous regression of cancer, and noninvasive treatment of cancer and cirrhosis of the liver.

Illness Treated

Various kinds of cancer, especially bone, breast, liver, ovarian, and colon; also cirrhosis of the liver and chronic hepatitis.

Treatment Offered

Local and systemic immuno-thermo-chemotherapy; sensitized lymphocyte therapy; LAK therapy; plasma exchange; herbal medicine; enhancement of natural healing power by use of refreshment therapy; and psychoimmunomodulation.

Related Readings

"Prospective Investigation of Tumor Markers and Risk Assesment in Early Cancer Screening." *Cancer*, Vol. 73, 1946-1953, 1994.

"New Primary Cancer Prevention. Methods of Risk Assessment Using a Tumor Marker Combination Assay." *Health Tactics in the 21st Century*, 327-330, 1994.

Length of Treatment/Stay

According to the degree or advanced situation of the disease, usually from three to eighteen months.

Costs

Varies according to the degree or advanced situation of the disease, usually from $6,000 U.S.*

Method of Payment

Cash only is accepted.

*Subject to the value of the U.S. dollar abroad.

Hufeland Klinik for Holistic Immunotherapy

Loeffelstelzer Str. 1-3
D-97980 Bad Mergentheim
Germany

011-49-7931-5360
Fax: 011-49-793-8185

Contact Person

Mrs. Bankoff; Mrs. Woeppel.

Primary Personnel

Wolfgang Woeppel, M.D., medical superintendent.

Directions

Take a plane to Frankfurt airport. From there, you can take a train or a taxi for the ninety miles southeast to Bad Mergentheim.

Background

The clinic offers a holistic concept tailored to the individual needs of each patient. The clinic follows the theory that a tumor is only the late-stage symptom of cancer, which is from the beginning a systemic disease caused by impaired functioning of the body's own defense and repair mechanisms. Cancer is not merely the disorder of one organ but is an expression of a comprehensive disorder of the whole person in his or her unity of body and soul. Traditional European naturopathy, empirical medicine, and conventional scientific medicine can be selectively used in a way that rebuilds people instead of destroying them. In case of treatment all doctor's reports, laboratory findings, and X-rays are needed. For special questions, call Dr. Woeppel at 011-49-7931-5360; the best chances to reach him are on Mondays, Thursdays, and Fridays, at 12 p.m. or Tuesdays at 6 p.m. German time (6 a.m. and 12 a.m. Eastern Standard Time), or send a fax to: 011-49-7931-46244.

Illness Treated

Malignant diseases of all kinds, especially breast cancer; melanoma; prostate, colon, and kidney cancer; brain tumors; and sarcomas. Also, chronic degenerative diseases, arthritis, indigestion, chronic fatigue syndrome, and arteriosclerosis. Also patients who have undergone or will soon undergo surgery, and want to strengthen their defenses before or after the operation. Treatment is not possible for acute leukemia or acute infectious diseases. The clinic does not accept patients who are confined to bed. Patients must not be too weak, and must be able to walk unaided.

Treatment Offered

Treatment includes specific and nonspecific attacks against tumors. Nonspecific treatments including regeneration of the organism by stimulating detoxifying functions of liver, kidneys, and intestines with the unique healing springs of Bad Mergentheim, further with colonics, and regeneration of the intestinal flora; eumetabolic therapy with homeopathic medicines, vitamins, minerals, enzymes, multistep oxygen therapy, ozone therapy, hydrogen peroxide therapy, chelation therapy, hydrotherapy, acupuncture, and nutrition; strengthening the body's natural defense mechanisms through immunotherapy with active fever, thymus extract, curative serums, interferon, infusions with mistletoe and echinacea preparations; biological response modifiers; and psychological treatment to strengthen the patient's will to recover with interviews, visualization, and relaxation methods. Specific treatments include careful low-dose chemotherapy, hormone therapy, or damaging certain subcutaneous tumors by electrogalvanic electricity. Pain treatment and full diagnostic methods are part of the program.

Length of Treatment/Stay

Four to eight weeks, depending on the individual. During the treatment, the patient is adjusted to the therapy, which can be continued at home with the help of a general practitioner.

Costs

Inpatients: 450 deutsche marks per day, which covers board, medicine, laboratory tests, doctor's consultations, and single room with shower. Outpatients: 370 deutsche marks per day, which covers medicine, laboratory tests, and doctor's consultations. If other medical services are necessary, such as consultations with other specialists, scans, or hospitalization, those who perform the service will bill the patient directly and separately.

Method of Payment

An 8,000 deutsche marks deposit is required upon arrival. Cash in deutsche marks and U.S. traveler's checks are the only methods accepted. Inquire with your own health insurance company for possible coverage of part or all of the cost of treatment.

Institute for Immunology and Thymus Research
(Institut fur Immunologie und Thymusforschung)

Rudolf-Huch-Str. 14
D-38667 Bad Harzburg
Germany

011-49-5322-960541
Fax: 011-49-5322-3017

Contact Person

Dr. Nicola Spiggelkotter.

Primary Personnel

Milan C. Pesic, M.D.

Directions

Fly to Frankfurt or Hannover airports. Bad Harzburg is approximately a one-hour ride from Hannover and approximately three hours from Frankfurt. A train (ICE) also goes from Hannover and Frankfurt to Bad Harzburg.

Background

THX/Thymex-L, a thymus extract, has been used in the treatment of more than 1.5 million patients in Europe, the United States, and Canada. It is an important immune modulator and immune corrector.

Illness Treated

Cancer; the best responders are lung, bladder, colon, pancreatic, and breast cancer, Hodgkin's disease, non-Hodgkin's lymphoma, and Kaposi's sarcoma. The institute also treats chronic degenerative diseases, including rheumatoid arthritis and lupus erythematosus (LES). Also accepted are patients who have metastatic cancer after having received an operation, radiation therapy, or chemotherapy.

Treatment Offered

THX/Thymex-L. It can be combined with other medicines. A diet is not necessary. After the first injections, it is possible that itching, redness, or swelling can occur locally; that should be treated with ointment. Other side effects are unknown. It is preferred that the patient first prepare general information about him- or herself, documentation of the illness, and details of the treatments received before. It is also preferred for the patient to send all the information and medical reports to the institute ahead of time, either by mail or fax. Office hours are Monday to Friday, except on Wednesday afternoon, 9 a.m. to 12 p.m. and 3 p.m. to 5 p.m. (German time). Full accommodations for the patient and accompanying persons are available at the clinic.

Related Readings

Experiences and Experimental Results with Whole Thymus Extract THX by Milan C. Pesic, M.D. Thymus Medizinischer Fachbuchverlag, Bad Harzburg, 1986.

"Therapeutic Possibilities of Thymic Preparations" by Milan C. Pesic, M.D. *A New Dimension in Scientific Research*, Vol. 1, No. 5:9-19, Washington.

"THX (Gesamt-Thymus-Extrakt nach Sandberg) bei der primar chronischen Polyarthritis und Gonarthrose" by Milan C. Pesic, M.D. *Erfahrungsheilkunde*, Bd. 31, Heft 10:790-796, Haug Verlag, Heidelberg, 1982.

Thymus—Zentrale der Immunitat und Endokrines Steuerungsorgan by Milan C. Pesic, M.D. Haug Verlag, Heidelberg, 1987.

Thymus Therapy—Selected Summaries and Brief Reports by Milan C. Pesic, M.D. Thymus Medizinischer Fachbuchverlag, Bad Harzburg, 1984.

Immunotherapie mit Thymusextrakt (THX) by Milan C. Pesic, M.D. Haug Verlag, Heidelberg, 1988.

Thymuspeptide, Thymusenzyme, Thymushormone in Forschung und Therapie by Milan C. Pesic (ed.), Thymus Medizinischer Fachbuchverlag, 1992.

Length of Treatment/Stay

Four to six weeks for cancer; one to three weeks for rheumatoid arthritis. Longer stays are available and are sometimes recommended, depending on the health status of the patient.

Costs

Treatment: $650 U.S., including all lab fees, blood and urine analyses, and medicine. Accommodations: $600 U.S. per week in the clinic. Accompanying persons: $600 U.S.* per week.

Method of Payment

Cash, money orders, and traveler's checks are accepted. Payment must be made two weeks in advance.

---

* Subject to the value of the U.S. dollar abroad.

Dr. Helmut Keller

(Chronic Disease Control and Treatment Center)

Am Reuthlein 2
D-95138 Bad Steben,
Germany

011-49-9288-5166
Fax: 011-49-9267-1040
Fax: 011-49-9288-7815

Primary Personnel

Dr. Helmut Keller.

Directions

The center is located in northeast Bavaria in the heart of the Franconian Forest.

Background

Dr. Keller offers a broad, individualized therapy based on monitoring the immune system. The Carnivora protocol is derived from the pressed juices of *Dionaea muscipula* plants, which are processed into a standardized pharmaceutical medication. Through continuing research over a period of twenty years, the treatment has been refined.

Illness Treated

Cancer, multiple sclerosis, chronic polyarthritis, Crohn's disease, ulcerative colitis, neurodermatitis, chronic viral diseases, immune deficiency, and auto-aggressive diseases.

Treatment Offered

Complete immune status evaluation; individualized treatments according to laboratory results and risks; preventative program; program before and after tumor operation designed to prevent metastases; use of copper, zinc, selenium, magnesium, lithium, vitamin C, vitamin E, beta-carotene, hyperthermia, and continual monitoring during treatment.

Length of Treatment/Stay

Patients are treated Monday through Friday for three to four hours per day. There is a recommended stay of four to six weeks, after which the patient can be released to the referring physician with a suggested treatment schedule.

Costs

Treatment, room, and board for four weeks: 10,000 to 12,000 deutsche marks. HIV patients receive Carnivora only; their four-week cost would be 8,000 to 10,000 deutsche marks, plus additional medication.

Method of Payment

Prepayment by traveler's or cashier's checks is accepted.

Hans A. Nieper, M.D.

Outpatient Office:
Sedan Strasse 21
30161 Hannover
Germany

011-0511-3-48-08-08 or 011-0511-3-31111
Fax: 011-0511-318417

Inpatient Clinic:
Paracelsus Klinik at Silbersee
Oertzeweg 24
30851 Langenhagen
Germany

Contact Person

Nurse Monica Malchert; Mrs. Otte (office); Mrs. Koch (hospital).

Primary Personnel

Hans Nieper, M.D., director of department of medicine.

Directions

Hannover is north of Frankfurt.

Background

Dr. Nieper is the founder of the German Society of Medical Tumor Therapy, and he researched electrolyte carriers (mineral transporters), which led to the development of his eumetabolic therapy. In 1972, he founded a deshielding therapy as well. He was president of the German Society of Oncology from 1982 to 1985. Outpatients see Dr. Nieper at his office. It is necessary to make reservations. Call from 9 a.m. to 4 p.m. (German time), preferably at 9 a.m., for an appointment. Confirm the appointment by letter. You can stay in a nearby hotel. For the inpatient program, you will stay at the hospital in Silbersee. Call from noon to 4 p.m. (German time) for reservations. Confirm by letter. Guests or companions can stay in a nearby hotel or in a private room or guest house. Bring along a tape recorder. For travel and hotel reservations, please contact United Airlines. Reservations can also be made by the office, 011-0511-3-48-08-08 or fax 011-0511-31-84-17, Nurse Monica Malchert or Mrs. Chr. Otte.

Illness Treated

Cancer, multiple sclerosis, arteriosclerosis, coronary disease, amyotrophic lateral sclerosis, rheumatoid arthritis, and osteoporosis.

Treatment Offered

Eumetabolic therapy at early stages of cancer. Therapy includes direct treatment of tumors (one way is with gene repair); improvement and restoration of the body's defenses; immune status assessment; and overcoming the blocking and shielding phenomenon. Other therapeutic tools used are beta-carotene, dialdehydes, squalene-ascorbate, ureylmandelonitrile, and enzymes.

Related Readings

A list of all Dr. Nieper's publications can be obtained from Brewer Science Library, Richland Center, Wisconsin 53581, United States, telephone (608) 647-6513. Materials are in German, Spanish, French, and English. One of his books is *Dr. Nieper's Revolution in Technology, Medicine, and Society.*

Length of Treatment/Stay

Depends on the health of the individual, but generally about eight to fourteen days. An appointment is required.

Costs

Outpatient therapy: approximately $1,500 U.S.,* but costs vary. Inpatient therapy: 450 to 550 deutsche marks per day, which includes the doctor's fee and all treatment costs. May be more with severe illness. Deposit is required.

Method of Payment

All bills are to be paid in cash (deutsche marks) or United States traveler's checks (but only in deutsche marks). Private insurance has been reimbursing 75 percent on the average.

---

* Subject to the value of the U.S. dollar abroad.

Optimum Health Centre

54-58 Jardine's Bazaar
Prosperous Commercial Building, 2nd Floor
Causeway Bay
Hong Kong

011-(852)-2577-3798
Fax: 011-(852)-2890-8469

Contact Person

Della Mak, manager.

Primary Personnel

Alexander Yuan, B.A., D.C., N.D., D.Ht.

Directions

The centre is located in the heart of Hong Kong's busiest shopping centre—Causeway Bay. The centre is easily accessible by all forms of public transportation—railway, bus, tram, mini-bus, and taxi, and within walking distance from several major hotels.

Background

Dr. Alexander Yuan received his undergraduate education in the United States. He then received his Doctor of Chiropractic degree from the Canadian Memorial Chiropractic College in 1982, his Doctor of Naturopathy from the Ontario College of Naturopathic Medicine (now the Canadian College of Naturopathic Medicine) in 1986, then further training in classical homeopathy, culminating in a diploma from a homeopathic college in India in 1987. He returned to Hong Kong in 1987 and established the Optimum Health Centre, which has become the oldest and largest natural health centre in Hong Kong. The centre offers a wide variety of analytic and healing systems and treatment modalities, and emphasizes a holistic approach to health care for the whole family. Regular lectures are conducted to educate the patients and their families on how to look after their health care needs.

Illness Treated

A full range of health problems, including cancers and AIDS.

Treatment Offered

Level One: symptoms/conditions treatment; Level Two: constitutional improvement; Level Three: anti-aging. A general constitutional program involves: gastrointestinal tract cleansing with colon hydrotherapy, herbal and nutritional supplements; improving blood quality with constitutional hydrotherapy; metabolic balancing with ionic therapy, utilizing urine and saliva testing according to Dr. Ream's equation of life; rebuilding digestion and tissue health with enzymes, herbs, and supplements; and dietary and lifestyle modifications.

Related Readings

The centre publishes a bilingual newsletter. Dr. Yuan is the author of two Chinese books and four audio tapes on natural healing. He also writes regular columns on natural medicine for several local magazines and newspapers. The health shop at the centre has the largest collection of books on natural healing for sale in Hong Kong.

Length of Treatment/Stay

This varies for different conditions and individual requirements. A minimum of six months is generally recommended for the constitutional program.

Costs

Initial consultation for general conditions is HK$300 to HK$800. For cancer conditions, HK$2,000, which includes fee to the cancer consultant. Follow-up consultation: HK$200 to HK$400. Total costs vary depending on the length of treatment and extent of program involved. Example of fees for different services include: live cell analysis, HK$400; ionic therapy test, HK$500; colonics, HK$400; hydrotherapy, HK$250.

Method of Payment

Patients pay by cash, check, or Visa, as service is rendered. Patients with insurance coverage pay the centre first, then claim their expenses from their insurance coverage with the receipts from the centre. The centre will not bill the insurance company.

Paracelsus Klinik

Center for Holistic Medicine and Dentistry
CH-9062 Lustmuehle
Switzerland

011-41-71-335-71-71
Fax: 011-41-71-335-71-00

Contact Person

Ulrich Schelling, administrative director.

Primary Personnel

Thomas Rau, M.D., medical director.

Background

The Center for Holistic Medicine and Dentistry was founded in 1958. It offers treatment of chronic diseases strictly applying natural methods and remedies.

Illness Treated

Cancer, chronic stomach and colon disturbances, cardiovascular disorders, chronic fungi problems, candida, intoxication, amalgam problems, and neuralgics.

Treatment Offered

Integrated tumor therapy: isopathy, terrain therapy according to Professor Enderlein, neural therapy, holistic biological tumor therapy including local and systemic hyperthermia, acid-base therapies, chelation therapy, orthomolecular therapy, elimination of toxic afflictions, and immune stimulation.

Length of Treatment/Stay

Treatment of cancer usually lasts about three weeks at the clinic. Post-treatment at a local doctor according to Paracelsus guidelines must be granted.

Costs

$200 to $300 U.S.* per day, not including accommodations.

Method of Payment

Cash, traveler's checks, and Visa are accepted. The clinic has no agreement with foreign insurance carriers, but does have an agreement with the Swiss Health Insurance System.

---

*Subject to the value of the U.S. dollar abroad.

Park Attwood Clinic

Trimpley, Bewdley
Worcestershire
DY12 1RE
England
United Kingdom

011-02997-444
Fax: 011-02997-375

Contact Person

Stephen Moore, administrator.

Primary Personnel

Dr. Maurice Orange; Dr. Frank A. Mulder.

Background

Park Attwood is registered under the English nursing home system for twelve beds. The two doctors are supported by a team of ten registered nurses, three artistic therapists, and two masseurs. The doctors prescribe mainly anthroposophical (homeopathy-based) medicines but will prescribe allopathic medicines where appropriate.

Illness Treated

Cancer in its many forms, rheumatic conditions, nervous system afflictions (particularly multiple sclerosis), and all forms of anxiety-related conditions (from life crises to mild forms of psychosis).

Treatment Offered

The regimen at Park Attwood begins with consultations with the doctors, who, in addition to prescribing medicines, are able to choose artistic therapy (painting, sculpture, and movement), rhythmical or hauschke massage, and speech therapy. Diet and the social life in the house provide support to the overall treatment.

Related Readings

Extending the Art of Healing by Dr. Michael R. Evans.

Anthroposophical Medicine by Victor Bott, M.D.

Anthroposophically Orientated Medicine and Its Remedies by Otto Wolff. Mercury Press, Spring Valley.

Length of Treatment/Stay

The average stay is three to six weeks.

Costs

Park Attwood operates on a policy of admission by medical need. Health insurance companies pay £130 per day for patients with policies who stay at Park Attwood. Otherwise, financial arrangements are made by individual negotiation. Park Attwood has recently introduced its own contribution scheme, the Park Attwood Patient Plan.

Method of Payment

Payment in any form should be received within thirty days of date of discharge. Checks drawn on banks from outside the United Kingdom are acceptable but will result in a 1 percent fee to cover bank charges.

EDUCATIONAL CENTERS

Institutes, Organizations, Physicians, Health Practitioners
North America (United States)

Pearl Bennette-Atkin, R.N., M.A., C.S.

85 Aspinwall Road
P.O. Box 950
Briarcliff Manor, New York 10510
United States

(914) 941-8926

170 West 81st Street
Suite 2D
New York, New York 10024
United States

(800) 473-6812

Primary Personnel

Pearl Bennette-Atkin, R.N., M.A., C.S.; Adam Atkin, Ph.D.

Background

This private consultation is offered as an adjunct to traditional or alternative medical therapies. Whatever medical treatment the patient has had or is now having, these therapies can help the patient to participate more actively in the healing process and enhance his or her life.

Illness Addressed

Cancer and all life-threatening and/or chronic debilitating illnesses.

Type of Program Offered

Private consultations include psychotherapy, holistic health counseling, and lifestyle recommendations. Also relaxation, visual imagery work, and shiatsu massage. Kinesiology and herbal recommendations are included.

Related Readings

Love, Medicine and Miracles by Bernie S. Siegel, M.D. Harper & Row, 1986
Healing Into Life and Death by Stephen Levine. Anchor/Doubleday, 1987.
You Can Heal Your Life by Louise Hay. Hay House, 1984
Healing Dimensions by Louis J. Marx, M.D. Neo-Paradigm Publishers.

Costs

Private consultations (including psychotherapy, relaxation, and body work): $50 to $75 per hour.

Method of Payment
Cash, checks, Visa, and MasterCard are accepted

Center for the Improvement of Human Functioning International, Inc.

3100 North Hillside
Wichita, Kansas 67219
United States

(316) 682-3100
Fax: (316) 682-5054
Internet: http://www.brightspot.org

Primary Personnel
Hugh Riordan, M.D.; Dr. Ron Hunninghake, M.D.

Directions
Highway 96 (NorthEast Expressway) to Hillside Avenue.

Background
The Center for the Improvement of Human Functioning International began in 1975 as a small nutritional research/clinical laboratory with a staff of three. Today, the center, also known as the Bright Spot for Health, is a complex medical, research, and educational organization with four major divisions: Olive W. Garvey Center for Healing Arts, Bio-Center Laboratory, Bio-Medical Synergistics Education Institute, and Bio-Communications Research Institute.

Illness Addressed
Any illness that has not adequately responded to standard medical care.

Type of Program Offered
A comprehensive biochemical, nutritional, energy, and mental medicine evaluation.

Related Readings
The center has numerous books, audio, and video tapes for sale.

Length of Program/Stay
One- to three-day evaluation.

Costs

The comprehensive history packet and initial office consultation and evaluation is $395 (children under 16, $295). The usual fees for laboratory testing may be in the range of $1,200 or more. Second appointment, about three weeks after evaluation, $85. Three subsequent appointments at one-month intervals, $50 each.

Method of Payment

Cash, personal checks, Visa, MasterCard, American Express, and Discover are accepted. The center files insurance for Medicare patients only. It will provide statements to the patient for filing insurance. Payment is expected at time of service.

The Chopra Center for Well Being

7630 Fay Avenue
La Jolla, California 92037
United States

(619) 551-7788
Fax: (619) 551-9570

Contact Person

Stephen Bickel, M.D., M.P.H., director.

Primary Personnel

David Simon, M.D., medical director.

Directions

Take 5 freeway, exit La Jolla Village Drive. Go west to Torrey Pines Road, turn left. Follow to end (Girard Street), and turn left. At next light, turn right. Next street is Fay; turn right.

Background

The center opened in August 1996. It provides mind-body educational programs and treatments for the enhancement of health and well-being. There are three medical doctors on staff. The center also has a cafe and a bookstore.

Illness Addressed

Cancer, coronary artery disease, chronic fatigue syndrome, AIDS, leukemia and other myeloprolific diseases, inflammatory diseases, irritable bowel syndrome, and anxiety and depression.

Type of Program Offered

Ayurvedic Panchakarma therapy (various massages, heat and herbal treatments, combined with special diets and herbal enemas); instruction in yoga, meditation, and nutrition; emotional workshops; visualization techniques; and evaluations by physicians trained in Ayurveda, internal medicine, family practice, and neurology.

Related Readings

Numerous books by Deepak Chopra: *Ageless Body; Timeless Mind; Quantum Healing; Seven Spiritual Laws of Success; Creating Health; Perfect Health; Journey Into Healing.*

Length of Program/Stay

Seven days.

Costs

$2,900 for the full seven-day package. Includes: medical and nurse consultations, seven days of Panchakarma therapy, meditation instruction, yoga classes, and all meals. Does not include lodging.

Method of Payment

Cash, checks, and credit cards are accepted. Insurance is not accepted.

Creative Health Institute

918 Union City Road
Union City, Michigan 49094
United States

(517) 278-6260
(517) 278-5837
Fax: (517) 278-7356

Contact Person

Donald O. Haughey.

Directions

Union City is south of Battle Creek. Take Coldwater Road east out of Union City. It becomes Union City Road heading southeast. The institute is in Hodunk halfway between Coldwater and Union City.

Background

Creative Health Institute is directly affiliated with the Ann Wigmore Foundation. The institute teaches a "living foods" lifestyle and offers people an opportunity to learn in a hands-on program. The ultimate goal of the center is to help people help themselves in body, mind, and spirit. The center is situated on 300 acres along the banks of the Coldwater River. This particular center has been open for fifteen years and can accommodate up to twenty people.

Illness Addressed

The center aims at achieving wellness through a living foods lifestyle. The center welcomes people who are able to care for themselves. If people are unable to do this, they may bring someone to tend to their physical needs. Guests and companions pay the regular program price. The center is not in a position to accept bed-ridden guests.

Type of Program Offered

The program practices remedial nutrition and consists of courses and lectures on different aspects of health and cleansing; there are daily exercise classes, relaxation periods, and educational videos available. A large part of the institute's focus is the hands-on experiential learning process addressing things such as sprouting, growing greens indoors, and living food preparation.

Related Readings

Be Your Own Doctor: A Positive Guide to Natural Living by Ann Wigmore. Avery Publishing Group, 1982.

Recipes for a Longer Life by Ann Wigmore. Avery Publishing Group, 1978.

The Sprouting Book by Ann Wigmore. Avery Publishing Group, 1986.

The Wheatgrass Book by Ann Wigmore. Avery Publishing Group, 1985.

Why Suffer? by Ann Wigmore. Avery Publishing Group, 1985.

The center also has a list of mail-order books.

Length of Program/Stay

The typical program length is two weeks. Discounts are available for longer stays.

Costs

Standard (dormitory) cost: $750 per program/$375 per week. Semiprivate: $950 per program/$475 per week. Private: $1,200 per program/$600 per week. All costs include classes/videos, meals, and accommodation.

Method of Payment

Cash, checks, and money orders are accepted.

Dale Figtree, Ph.D.

1605 Bath Street #1
Santa Barbara, California 93101
United States

(805) 963-9224

Illness Addressed

Degenerative diseases.

Type of Program Offered

Dr. Figtree offers concentrated nutritional programs directed at supporting and restoring the body's own ability to cleanse, repair, rebalance, and heal itself.

Related Readings

Health After Cancer by Dale Figtree, Ph.D.
Eat Smart by Dale Figtree, Ph.D.

Costs

$100 for first consultation, $75 for follow-up consultations.

George Ohsawa Macrobiotic Foundation

1999 Meyers Street
Oroville, California 95966
United States

(916) 533-7702
(800) 232-2372 for orders or information requests.
Fax: (916) 533-7908

Contact Person

Herman and Cornellia Aihara, directors.

Primary Personnel

Carl Ferre, general manager; Laurel Ruggles, financial officer.

Directions

Please call.

Background

Over twenty-five years of providing macrobiotic education and support services.

Illness Addressed

All illnesses are addressed.

Type of Program Offered

Mail order macrobiotic book catalog. *Macrobiotics Today* magazine. French Meadows Summer Camp—ten days in Tahoe National Forest.

Related Readings

Over 175 books and videos.

Length of Program/Stay

Ten-day camp program.

Costs

$500 for members ($20 membership fee).

Method of Payment

Checks, cash, Visa, MasterCard, and American Express are accepted.

Gerson Therapy Self-Help

P.O. Box 16222
Oakland, California 94610
United States

(800) 851-8473 (leave message)
(510) 444-3689

Contact Person

Marilyn Barnes.

Primary Personnel

Marilyn Barnes.

Background

Marilyn is a seventeen-year recovered cancer patient (melanoma and cervical cancer) on the Gerson Therapy. She was the owner of the Gerson Halfway House—a long-term facility that offered the full Gerson Therapy of juices, organic meals, and support counseling for nine years. Marilyn has also participated in nutritional demonstrations, health seminars, and radio and TV interviews. She has been personal chef and a "living proof" testimonial for Gerson Institute Seminars and Charlotte Gerson. Her experience now includes helping many patients initiate and/or organize the Gerson Therapy in their homes.

Illness Addressed

Cancer, diabetes, arthritis, multiple sclerosis, AIDS, heart problems, allergies, and others.

Type of Program Offered

Marilyn travels to any location worldwide to assist individuals in starting or continuing the Gerson Therapy. She organizes the kitchen, teaches juicing and cooking methods, assists with food and equipment purchases, shows how to effectively budget time and money, helps with personal applications and support counseling, insures mistakes are not made, and demonstrates the preparation of tasty, gourmet Gerson meals.

Related Readings

A Cancer Therapy—Results of 50 Cases by Max Gerson, M.D.
Gerson Primer.
Cancer Winner by Jacquie Davidson.

Length of Program/Stay

Three days to two weeks.

Costs

Daily fee and transportation costs to be negotiated.

Method of Payment

Cash or money order is accepted.

Health Action

243 Pebble Beach
Santa Barbara, California 93117
United States

(805) 685-4670
(800) 824-4325

Contact Person

Dr. Roger Jahnke.

Primary Personnel

Roger Jahnke, O.M.D., Doctor of Acupuncture and Oriental Medicine; Rebecca McLean, director of health education.

Directions

The center is north of central Santa Barbara. Traveling on U.S. 101 for 100 miles from Los Angeles and 350 miles south of San Francisco, exit at Storke-Glen Annie Road. Go one block toward ocean, turn right on Hollister Road. Go one mile and turn left on Pebble Beach.

Background

Health Action has provided innovative services for people with chronic and life-threatening diseases for over fifteen years. The essence of Health Action's program is that the most profound medicine is produced within each person.

Illness Addressed

All cancer diagnoses and side effect syndromes; HIV/AIDS; and chronic fatigue.

Type of Program Offered

For those who are using conventional medical therapy, this program is complementary to the treatment. For those who elect natural healing, this program is cooperative with the patient's other healing choices. The center offers qi gong (chi kung), tai chi, yoga, meditation, cancer self-care, self-healing home program development, and a support group. Clinical services include acupuncture, massage, herbs, and homeopathy.

Related Readings

The Self-Applied Health Enhancement Methods by Roger Jahnke, O.M.D. Health Action Publishing.

The Most Profound Medicine by Roger Jahnke, O.M.D., Health Action Publishing.

Quigong-Chi kung: Awakening the Medicine Within. Health Action Publishing.

The Relaxation Response by Herbert Benson, M.D.

Encounters With Qi by David Eisenberg, M.D.

Length of Program/Stay

Varies with each patient.

Costs

Clinical visits: $80 to $100 first visit; $65 to $75 for additional visits. Support: $65 to $75; Group: $30 per person. Goals clarification: $65 to $75. Qi gong-chi kung workshop or retreat: $75 to $200.

Method of Payment

Cash, checks, Visa, and MasterCard are accepted. Many insurance companies cover portions of the programs. Get advanced approval. Health Action will provide receipt of the patient's payment, which then may be submitted for reimbursement.

HealthQuarters Lodge

P.O. Box 62130
Colorado Springs, Colorado 80962-2130
United States

(719) 593-8694
Fax: (719) 531-7884

Contact Persons

Jim Goodwin, C.E.O.; Sharon Brechtl, public relations/counselor.

Primary Personnel

Dave and Anne Frahm, founders; Sonia Mirza, certified nutritionist.

Background

In 1991, Dave and Anne Frahm wrote a book, *A Cancer Battle Plan*, detailing the nutritional approach that Anne had used to help win back her own health from the clutches of "terminal" breast cancer. The response they received from thousands of readers led them to launch HealthQuarters Lodge—an education and resource center for better health through nutrition. Today, people come from all over the country to participate in eleven-day sessions at the lodge in order to learn and begin to put into practice certain diet and lifestyle changes that will help them move toward improved health.

Illness Addressed

Primarily cancer, although many other chronic degenerative condtions will benefit from diet and lifestyle changes, including allergies, arthritis, heart and circulatory problems, diabetes, environmental illness, and lupus.

Type of Program Offered

Individualized nutritional assessment and evaluation; generalized detoxification education and experience; "live foods" diet classes; personal health care products education; health food store field trip; prayer power sessions and devotionals; mild exercise, relaxation, and massage; "going home" dietary plan; individually tailored plan of supplements; and networking information for ongoing professional help.

Related Readings

A Cancer Battle Plan by Dave and Anne Frahm. Pinon Press.

Healthy Habits by Dave and Anne Frahm. Pinon Press.

Reclaim Your Health by Dave and Anne Frahm. Pinon Press.

Raw, Raw, Raw by Dave and Anne Frahm. HealthQuarters Ministries.

A Cancer Therapy by Max Gerson, M.D. The Gerson Institute.

Beating Cancer with Nutrition by Patrick Quillin, Ph.D., R.D. Nutrition Times Press.

Nutrition: The Cancer Answer by Maureen Salaman. Statford Publishing.

One Answer to Cancer by W.D. Kelley, D.D.S. Wedgestone Press.

Cancer and Nutrition by Charles B. Simone, M.D. Avery Publishing Group.

Wellness Against All Odds by Sherry Rogers, M.D. Prestige Publishing.

God's Way to Ultimate Health by George Malkmus. Hallelujah Acres Publishing.

Coronary? Cancer? God's Answer: Prevent It! by Richard O. Brennan, M.D. Harvest House.

Cancer and Its Nutritional Therapies by Richard A. Passwater, Ph.D. Keats Publishing.

Prescription for Nutritional Healing by James Balch, M.D. and Phyllis Balch, C.N.C. Avery Publishing Group.

Costs

Please call for current information.

Method of Payment

Cash, checks, money orders, Visa, and MasterCard are accepted. Insurance does not cover this sort of nutrition-based program.

Hippocrates Health Institute

1443 Palmdale Court
West Palm Beach, Florida 33411
United States

(407) 471-8876
(800) 842-2125

Contact Person

Ask for program counselors or for reservations.

Primary Personnel

Brian and Anna Marie Clement, directors.

Directions

Take Florida Turnpike to Okeechobee exit (West Palm Beach). Turn right onto Okeechobee Road to second light (Skees Road). Turn left onto Skees and go three-quarters of a mile to Palmdale Road. Turn right; then take first right onto Palmdale Court. Go to the end of the street. The institute is ten minutes from West Palm Beach International Airport.

Background

For more than forty years, Hippocrates Health has pioneered the development of a lifestyle program of nutrition through living foods, moderate exercise, and stress reduction. The concept of living foods began in the United States with Ann Wigmore and a dedicated group of health pioneers. Through extensive research and experimentation, Hippocrates Health has continued to update its health restoration program, and today it enjoys a worldwide reputation among professionals and lay people. Its program consists of a cleansing and nourishing diet of live foods integrated with a range of holistic therapies. The program teaches a plan of gradual transition to a more healthful lifestyle that people can implement in their daily lives.

Illness Addressed

All types of cancer and degenerative diseases.

Type of Program Offered

The program includes a special diet consisting of uncooked vegetables, fresh fruits, sprouted seeds, grains, and beans. Wheatgrass juice therapy is usually prescribed. There are daily classes in exercise, human physiology, body purification, detoxification, food preparation, sprouting, and stress management. Also available are massages, electromagnetic treatments, an oxygenated pool, and a sauna, as well as the services of a professional nonresidential staff: medical doctor, dentist, colon therapist, chiropractor, psychologist, psychoneuroimmunology specialist, and aesthetician.

Related Readings

Be Your Own Doctor: A Positive Guide to Natural Living by Ann Wigmore. Avery Publishing Group, 1982.

Belief by Brian Clement. Hippocrates Publications, 1991.

The Hippocrates Diet and Health Program by Ann Wigmore. Avery Publishing Group, 1984.

How I Conquered Cancer Naturally by Eydie Mae Hunsberger. Avery Publishing Group.

The Wheatgrass Book by Ann Wigmore. Avery Publishing Group, 1985.

Hippocrates Health Program: A Proven Guide to Healthful Living by Brian Clement. Hippocrates Publications, 1990.

(The center will in some cases provide information regarding past patients.)

Length of Program/Stay

Three weeks recommended. Stays of one or two weeks are also available.

Costs

On-site accommodations range from $125 per day for a dormitory room to $300 per day for a private deluxe room. Costs include all meals, classes, activities, one massage per week, electromagnetic treatments, private consultations with the directors, live cell analysis, and clinical bloodwork. Some people may want to join the program but live off premises. Up to twelve such students will be admitted. Each nonresident student pays $2,900 for three weeks. Plus, for those with a trailer or mobile home, the Pine Lake Camp Resort for recreational vehicles is only minutes away.

Method of Payment

Money orders, cashier's checks, American Express, MasterCard, and Visa are accepted. Some insurance is accepted. To secure a place in the program, students must make reservations, either over the telephone by using one of the accepted credit cards or by mailing a nonrefundable deposit of half the total cost. Any balance due is payable upon arrival.

Hydeout

28195 Fairview Avenue
Hemet, California 92544
United States

(909) 927-1768
Fax: (909) 927-1548

Contact Person

Evarts G. Loomis, M.D.; Fay L. Loomis, M.A.

Primary Personnel

Evarts G. Loomis, M.D.; Fay L. Loomis, M.A.

Directions

Two hours southeast of Los Angeles, one hour west of Palm Springs, and two hours north of San Diego. From Hemet, take Fairview Avenue south to the end of the pavement. Continue about one mile on dirt road.

Background

Evarts and Fay Loomis counsel, write, and lecture internationally on holistic health. Evarts founded and operated Meadowlark, America's first holistic health retreat, from 1957 to 1991.

Illness Addressed

General and chronic conditions.

Type of Program Offered

Hydeout is a quiet retreat house where guests can set up their own program. Health consultation is offered, and a sizeable library of books and tapes on a holistic view of health and personal growth is available. The Hydeout, located on the 580-acre Friendly Hills Ranch, has trails into surrounding hills and canyons. Modalities include homeopathy, fasting, kinesiology, journaling, and dream work.

Length of Program/Stay

Usually, up to two consultations. Length of Hydeout stay determined by guest.

Costs

$150 for initial consultation; $75 for follow-up. $75 per day for Hydeout for one person; $100 for two; $125 for three. Last day is free for a weekly stay. Food is provided and prepared by guest.

Method of Payment

Checks or cash is accepted.

Izaac David Frees Organic Health Research

811 Summit Road
Santa Barbara, California 93108
United States

(805) 565-1080

Contact Person

Izaac David Frees.

Primary Personnel

Izaac David Frees, B.A., H.M., C.H.T., P.L.T., R.T.

Directions

Please call the office for directions.

Background

Izaac David Frees has twelve years' experience in research and consulting in the alternative and naturopathic fields. He uses primarily food and diet, rather than pills and supplements, to accomplish healing, regeneration, and detoxification.

Illness Addressed

Full range of degenerative diseases.

Type of Progam Offered

Full diet/food program, Reichian therapy, and colon hydrotherapy.

Related Readings

Nourishing Traditions by Sally Zallon.
Natural Foods Are Your Best Medicine by Dr. Ralph Schmid.
Alternative Medicine by the Goldberg Group.

Length of Program/Stay

Single consultation, followed by three to four months' detoxification consult and services.

Costs

Range from $60 to $90 per hour.

Method of Payment

Cash or checks are accepted. Insurance is not accepted.

Kushi Institute

P.O. Box 7
Becket, Massachusetts 01223
United States

(413) 623-5741

Primary Personnel

Michio Kushi.

Background

The Kushi Institute (a division of the Kushi Foundation) is directed by educators Michio and Aveline Kushi. The institute teaches a natural approach to health, based upon a whole foods diet and natural lifestyle. It has been used by countless individuals as a means of recovering from various illnesses, including cancer. Courses are offered in macrobiotic cooking for health, philosophy, macrobiotic health care, nutrition, and shiatsu massage. During the past seventeen years, the Kushis and their associates have developed a comprehensive approach to preventing and treating degenerative diseases. Research studies at Harvard Medical School, the Framingham Heart Study, Boston University, and elsewhere supported the value of the macrobiotic approach. In 1994, the Kushi Institute and the University of Minnesota were the recipients of a grant from the National Institutes of Health (NIH) to investigate the macrobiotic approach to cancer therapy. The Kushi Foundation and the Kushi Institute are not medical clinics, nor do they offer medical diagnosis or treatment. They offer education to persons interested in learning more about the natural, macrobiotic approach to health. The institute also has several locations in Europe.

Illness Addressed

Cancer, heart disease, diabetes, and AIDS, as well as any other health problem.

Type of Program Offered

The one-week program is recommended for those in a recovery process: *The Way to Health, Parts 1 and 2.* This program provides basic (Part 1) and more advanced (Part 2) information on the macrobiotic approach to health, including lectures, demonstrations, cooking classes, and, if requested, a private interview to adjust the macrobiotic diet to particular health needs. For those wanting in-depth studies, a one-month program, *Dynamics of Macrobiotics*, is offered. This program includes classes, Oriental diagnosis, philosophy, and shiatsu massage. This course is offered in three levels. Other week-long and weekend programs, from health recovery to gourmet macrobiotic cooking, are available.

Related Readings

The Cancer-Prevention Diet by Michio Kushi and Alex Jack. St. Martin's Press, 1985.

The Macrobiotic Approach to Cancer by Michio Kushi with Ed Esko. Second edition. Avery Publishing Group, 1991.

The Macrobiotic Cancer Prevention Cookbook by Aveline Kushi with Wendy Esko. Avery Publishing Group, 1988.

Macrobiotic Diet by Michio Kushi with Alex Jack. Tokyo: Japan Publications, 1985.

The Macrobiotic Way by Michio Kushi and Steven Blauer. Avery Publishing Group, 1985.

The Changing Seasons Macrobiotic Cookbook by Aveline Kushi and Wendy Esko. Avery Publishing Group, 1985.

Cancer Free by Ann Fawcett and the East/West Foundation.

These books and others, plus video and audio tapes, macrobiotic foods, and cookware, are available by mail order through the foundation.

Costs

$1,250 for week-long programs, $350 for weekend programs. Discounts are available.

Method of Payment

Checks, money orders, Visa, MasterCard, and American Express are accepted as payment through the mail.

Life Extension Nutrition Center

995 Southwest 24th Street
Fort Lauderdale, Florida 33315
United States

(800) 841-5433

P.O. Box 229120
Hollywood, Florida 33022-9120
United States

(954) 766-5433

Directions

From I-95, take State Road 84 (which is Southwest 24th Street) east one mile to Southland Shopping Plaza.

Background

This is a nonprofit organization dedicated to funding research in gerontology and providing people with information concerning living longer.

Illness Addressed

The center provides information on sources of alternative therapies for a variety of illnesses.

Type of Program Offered

The center does not offer any treatments, only information and referrals.

Related Readings

Life Extension by Durk Pearson and Sandy Shaw
Cancer Therapy by Ralph Moss.

Costs

Cost of supplements.

Method of Payment

Cash, checks, money orders, Visa, MasterCard, American Express, and Discover are accepted. The center does not accept insurance, but some insurance companies may cover vitamins.

Linus Pauling Institute

Oregon State University
571 Weniger Hall #15
Corvallis, Oregon 97331
United States

(541) 737-5075

Contact Person

Stephen Lawson, administrative officer.

Primary Personnel

Dr. Donald Reed, interim director; Stephen Lawson, administrative officer; Ober Tyus, development officer.

Background

The institute conducts basic research on important health concerns.

Illness Addressed

Research areas include cancer, cardiovascular disease, and degenerative diseases.

Type of Program Offered

The institute is an interdisciplinary research center at O.S.U. engaged in nutrition-oriented biomedical research. It does not maintain clinical facilities, and accordingly does not conduct treatment programs for patients. It does, however, offer information about its research and about the work and books by the late Nobelist Linus Pauling, and his colleague Ewan Cameron.

Related Readings

Cancer and Vitamin C by Ewan Cameron and Linus Pauling. Linus Pauling Institute of Science and Medicine, 1979. Updated and expanded, 1993.

How to Live Longer and Feel Better by Linus Pauling. 1986.

Costs

Tax-deductible donations.

Macrobiotic Centers

See George Ohsawa Macrobiotic Foundation, Kushi Institute, and Vega Study Center, all in this section. For more information about macrobiotic programs, see *International Macrobiotic Directory*, available by contacting Bob Mattson at 1050 40th Street, Oakland, California 94608, telephone (510) 601-1763. Another important resource is Health Classics (National Macrobiotic Educational Seminars), P.O. Box 30254, Santa Barbara, California 93130-0254, telephone (805) 898-0089 or fax (805) 898-1428.

Medical Health and Fitness

P.O. Box 29
Santa Barbara, California 93102
United States

(805) 884-8120
1074 Miramonte Drive #1
Santa Barbara, California 93109
United States

Contact Person

Eric P. Durak, M.Sc., director.

Background

Medical Health and Fitness is a research and consulting business whose primary mission is the integration of exercise and health promotion into health care. Since 1992, M.H.F. has promoted this concept via publications, seminars, and assistance in designing health care-based exercise facilities.

Illness Addressed

The main illnesses addressed are breast and prostate cancers and leukemia.

Type of Program Offered

Information centers on aerobic exercise, strength and conditioning, pain-free movement, and stress reduction, and their effects on cancer recovery.

Related Readings

Their book, *Cancer, Exercise, Wellness, and Rehab,* was published in the spring of 1996, and addresses all of the issues concerning exercise and lifestyle in cancer rehab and recovery.

Costs

Cost of the cancer book is $19.95 plus $3.00 shipping and handling. Other costs vary.

Method of Payment

Cash is accepted.

New Life Health Center

12 Harris Avenue
Jamaica Plain, Massachusetts 02130
United States

(617) 524-9551
Fax: (617) 524-0345

Primary Personnel

Bo-In Lee, licensed acupuncturist.

Directions

The New Life Health Center is located in the Jamaica Plain section of greater Boston, and is easily accessible by car and public transportation.

Background

The New Life Health Center was founded in 1980 by Bo-In Lee. Bo-In Lee was educated in Oriental medicine in his native Korea, Japan, and India, and came to the United States in 1977. He is a licensed acupuncturist, Zen meditation master, and yoga master. The center offers a Resident Healing Program as well as outpatient care for people with cancer and chronic illness. The underlying cause, seen as imbalance, and its accompanying physical, mental, emotional, and spiritual issues, are all addressed through an individually designed and integrated healing program to optimize immune power and achieve a state of homeostasis. The patient's own healing power is emphasized, as well as self-knowledge and a positive mental attitude.

Illness Addressed

All illnesses are treated. Most patients come with cancer and chronic illness.

Type of Program Offered

A Resident Healing Program of three weeks is recommended for those with cancer or serious chronic illness. Bo-In Lee uses the diagnostic findings of Western and Oriental medicine to design a treatment plan that may include, but is not limited to, acupuncture, moxibustion, cupping and herbal teas, nutritional therapy, and a supervised cleansing fast when indicated. Daily yoga and meditation classes are given weekdays, as well as educational lectures on healing and a healthy lifestyle. A natural, whole foods, grain-based diet including brown rice and miso soup is offered.

Related Readings

Wake Up! You Can Heal Yourself by Bo-In Lee, 1985.
The New Life Cancer Treatment by Bo-In Lee, 1994.

Length of Program/Stay

Individually determined. Average stay is three to six weeks.

Costs

Resident Healing Program: $995 per week with semi-private accommodations. $1,095 per week with private accommodations. Price includes room and meals, five daily treatments of Oriental medicine, one weekly treatment of psychological counseling, access to daily lectures, yoga and meditation classes, and a supervised cleansing fast, when indicated.

Method of Payment

Cash and checks are accepted. Upon request, receipted bills with a diagnosis are provided for patients to submit to their own insurance companies for reimbursement.

Optimum Health Institute of San Diego

6970 Central Avenue
Lemon Grove, California 91945
United States

(619) 464-3346
Fax: (619) 589-4098

Primary Personnel

Robert P. Nees, president, cofounder.

Background

This is a premiere holistic health center. The program is based on a 100-percent living foods diet to eliminate body toxins. There is an open house every Sunday at 4:30 p.m., for interested individuals. The facility has a maximum capacity of 200 guests. The program itself starts on Sundays.

Illness Addressed

Illnesses are not addressed. Emphasis is on wellness.

Type of Program Offered

Diet and exercise. The living foods diet includes: sprouts, greens, fruits, vegetables, enzymatic seed sauces, juices, enzyme-rich rejuvelac, sauerkraut, and wheatgrass juice. The facility also provides classes dealing with exercise, nutrition, positive thinking, food preparation, and emotional and spiritual development.

Related Readings

Survival Into the 21st Century by Viktoras Kulvinskas. Omangod Press, 1975.
Coming Alive with Raychel by Raychel Solomon and Dr. Mark Solomon.
Books, cassette tapes, and equipment to maintain a live foods lifestyle as it is taught in this program are available through mail order.

Length of Program/Stay

Three-week stays are recommended, but shorter stays of one or two weeks are accepted.

Costs

A $50 deposit per week of stay is required two weeks before arrival. Private room (standard): $475 per week. Double room: $325 per week per person. One-bedroom townhouse: $600 per week if just one person; $400 per person per week if two people. Executive suite: $600 per person/$900 per couple each week. Other accommodations are also available. This fee includes room, meals, linens, lectures, and classes, and is to be paid in full upon arrival. At extra cost are books and equipment.

Method of Payment

Cash, personal checks, traveler's checks, money orders, cashier's checks, MasterCard, Visa, and American Express are accepted.

Ray Peat, Ph.D.

P.O. Box 5764
Eugene, Oregon 97405
United States

(541) 345-9855

Contact Person

Raymond Peat, Ph.D.

Primary Personnel

Raymond Peat, Ph.D.

Background

Raymond Peat holds a Ph.D. in biology (biochemistry minor) from the University of Oregon, 1972. Dr. Peat is concerned with the interactions between environmental toxins, radiation, diet, and hormones. He publishes a monthly newsletter, *Ray Peat's Newsletter.*

Illness Addressed

Degenerative diseases.

Type of Program Offered

Research and education, with an endocrine and dietary approach. Special emphasis is placed on the thyroid, progesterone, and pregnenolone.

Related Readings

Generative Energy.

Mind and Tissue.

Nutrition for Women.

Progesterone in Orthomolecular Medicine.

Ray Peat's Newsletter.

Length of Program/Stay

One day per week.

Costs

$80 per hour of consultation.

Method of Payment

Checks are acceptable.

Southeast Research Foundation Inc.

5416 Glen Cove Drive
Knoxville, Tennessee 37919
United States

(423) 588-7678
(423) 584-8150

Contact Person

Chris Poole, treasurer.

Background

The foundation was founded in 1983 by Dr. Cecil Pitard, who was stricken with cancer in 1981 and given a prognosis of six months to live. He developed a protocol for the treatment of cancer and applied it to himself, adding another ten years to his life.

Illness Addressed

All types of cancer; good responses with leukemia, bone cancer, and brain tumors; but any other cancer—including breast cancer—can respond well, too, depending upon an individual's biochemistry and state of health.

Type of Program Offered

The foundation identifies and explains the use of Dr. Pitard's protocol of all-natural drugs and vitamins, some taken orally and others by injection. Information is offered to patients, doctors, and other interested parties. The foundation does not dispense the drugs, some of which require a physician's prescription. In all cases, a doctor's supervision is recommended. The patient will likely know within a month of being on the full program (taking all drugs prescribed) whether it will help.

Costs

The foundation is a nonprofit organization and does not charge any fees. However, donations are welcome. Patients can purchase ingredients for the protocol for less than $3 per day of treatment.

Syracuse Cancer Research Institute Inc.

Presidential Plaza
600 East Genesee Street
Syracuse, New York 13202
United States

(315) 472-6616

Primary Personnel

Joseph Gold, M.D.

Background

Founded by its director, Dr. Joseph Gold, the institute began operations at its present location early in 1966. At the time, the cause of cancer cachexia—the weight loss and debilitation seen in cancer patients—was unknown. Dr. Gold found that the condition is largely the result of cancer's ability to "recycle wastes" at the energy expense of the body, thus imposing a severe energy drain on the body. Specifically, it was pointed out that cancer uses glucose (sugar) as its fuel but metabolizes it incompletely. Hydrazine sulfate is one of a new class of gluconeogenic blocking agents that functions as a specific chemotherapeutic agent for cancer cachexia. The drug, developed by the Syracuse Cancer Research Institute, has been in limited clinical use since late 1973. This substance, based on the work of Dr. Gold, and seventeen years of testing via the joint U.S.-U.S.S.R. Cancer Commission, is now an approved first-line cancer drug in Russia. It is undergoing further testing in the United States with National Cancer Institute sponsorship.

Illness Addressed

Cancer.

Type of Program Offered

Your doctor can write to the institute and receive an information packet for physicians; it includes reports on tests with hydrazine sulfate.

Related Readings

"Proposed Treatment of Cancer by Inhibition of Gluconeogenesis" by Joseph Gold, M.D. *Oncology* 22, pages 185-207, 1968.

"Use of Hydrazine Sulfate in Terminal and Preterminal Cancer Patients: Preliminary Results" (abstr.) by Joseph Gold, M.D., *Proc Am Assoc Cancer Res* 15, 83, 1974'.

"Hydrazine Sulfate Influence on Nutritional Status and Survival in Non-Small-Cell Lung Cancer" by Roan T. Debowski, et al. *Journal of Clinical Oncology.* 8:9-15, 1990.

"Treatment of Primary Brain Tumors with Sehydrin (Hydrazine Sulfate)" by V.A. Filov, et al. *Probl Oncol* 40:332-336, 1994.

Costs

Contributions to the cash fund are accepted. Contributions of equities are placed in the cash fund or in the endowment fund, depending on the donor's wishes. All contributions are tax-deductible.

Method of Payment

Checks and money orders are accepted.

Vega Study Center

1511 Robinson Street
Oroville, California 95965
United States

(916) 533-4777
(800) 818-VEGA
Fax: (916) 533-4999

Contact Person

Herman and Cornellia Aihara, directors.

Primary Personnel

David Briscoe, manager.

Directions

Take Highway 70 one hour and fifteen minutes north of Sacramento.

Background

The center has offered macrobiotic programs since 1974. These programs include: cancer and healing, vital immunity, and diabetes and hypoglycemia.

Illness Addressed

All, especially cancer.

Type of Program Offered

Macrobiotic approach.

Related Readings

Natural Healing from Head to Toe by Herman and Cornellia Aihara. Avery Publishing Group, 1994.

Essential Ohsawa by George Ohsawa. Avery Publishing Group, 1994.

Acid and Alkaline by Herman Aihara.

Basic Macrobiotic Cooking by Julia Ferre.

Calendar Cookbook by Cornellia Aihara.

Length of Program/Stay

One, two, or three weeks.

Costs

Approximately $500 per week, plus accommodations.

Method of Payment

Cash, checks, Visa, MasterCard, and American Express are accepted.

Wellness Center Associates, Inc.

5757 Wilshire Boulevard, Suite 2
Los Angeles, California 90036
United States

(213) 464-4141
Fax: (213) 464-8979

Contact Person

Dr. Rene Espy; Dr. Nancy McBride.

Primary Personnel

Chiropractors; massage therapist.

Directions

Wilshire between Fairfax and LaBrea.

Background

Dr. Rene Espy received a Doctor of Chiropractic degree from Texas Chiropractic College. She is the clinic director of Wellness Center Associates, and conducts seminars for doctors throughout the United States, Canada, and Europe on current research relating to major breakthroughs in alternative health care and the immune system.

Illness Addressed

Neuromuscular skeletal disorders, muscular dystrophy, polio, post-polio, strokes, Charcot-Marie-Tooth atrophy, and the immune system.

Type of Program Offered

Total body care, nutrition, chiropractic, and kinesiology.

Length of Program/Stay

Two to three weeks. Three hours per day for out-of-town patients.

Costs

$200 per hour.

Method of Payment

Cash, checks, and credit cards are accepted.

Writers and Research Inc.

4810 St. Paul Boulevard
Rochester, New York 14617
United States

(716) 266-4630
Fax: (716) 544-1838
E-mail: pix@frontiernet.net

Contact Person

Charles or Judy Pixley

Primary Personnel

Charles Pixley, president; Dr. Dietmar Schildwaechater, M.D., Ph.D., institutional review board chief investigator.

Background

First institutional review board set up under the laws of Congress by an independent citizen to coordinate FDA approval, educate the American public, and obtain informed consent from those pursuing treatment with the camphor-based homeopathic medicinal called 714X, representing the research of Gaston Naessens.

Illness Addressed

Cancer, viral, and degenerative diseases.

Type of Program Offered

714X, an immune function stabilizer, proteolytic enzyme therapy as originally designed in the 1930s by Doctors Gaschler, Wolf, and Benitez, founders of WoBe Mucos, WoBenzyme. 714X and enzymes are self-administered. Complete information is provided to patient or professional on the correct use of these therapies. A blood test, which is highly calibrated to prediagnose cancer two years before clinical manifestations, is given.

Related Readings

The Persecution and Trial of Gaston Naessens by Christopher Bird. H.J. Kramer, Inc., 1991.

Length of Program/Stay

Minimum recommended therapy is six months, and may last up to two years depending on the severity and extent of activity or degeneration.

Costs

Six-month combination metabolic therapy, which includes 714X, proteolytic enzyme therapy, and two blood tests: $5,500, payable by the month.

Method of Payment

Cash, checks, money orders, Visa, and MasterCard are accepted.

EDUCATIONAL CENTERS

Institutes, Organizations, Physicians, Health Practitioners
Overseas (Australia, Japan, New Zealand, United Kingdom)

I. J. Bullen

297 Pearson Street
Woodlands
Western Australia 6018
Australia

011-09-4451994

Contact Person
Surgery receptionist.

Primary Personnel
I.J. Bullen, M.B.B.S., D.Obst. R.C.O.G., and Dr. J. Han, Ph.D.

Directions
Take Mitchell Freeway northbound, exit at Powis Street, go straight ahead to Jon Sanders Drive. After passing through an industrial area, Jon Sanders Drive changes name to Pearson Street. The doctor's office is on the right, three houses before the Leige Street traffic lights. (Because of a median strip, you will need to go past the lights, turn around, and come back again.)

Background
Dr. Bullen is a general practitioner with an interest in the supportive care of cancer patients through meditation, counseling, nutrition, and four-day health retreats. Dr. Bullen is a member of the Australian College of Nutritional and Environmental Medicine. Dr. Han is a psychologist whose clientele includes many cancer patients. He is a member of the Australian Psychological Society.

Illness Addressed
Cancer.

Type of Program Offered
General medical care, nutritional advice, intravenous vitamin C, counseling, meditation, allergy assessment, and four-day health retreats. The retreats are held in fully equipped log cabins in a beautiful bushland setting in Jarrahdale Hills (about forty-five minutes from the city). Each retreat commences Thursday morning and concludes late Sunday afternoon. The program covers medical, psychological, and nutritional areas. Topics such as therapeutic massage, Reiki, and other complementary approaches are also included. To balance the holistic program, an oncologist and a radiotherapist speak on their specialties and on the structure and function of the

immune system. In an informal, relaxed setting, patients often find answers to many of their difficult questions. All meals are vegetarian and low in fat, and are as close to 100 percent organic as the staff can manage.

Related Readings

Man the Healer by Jose Silva.

Cancer and Vitamin C by Linus Pauling and Ewan Cameron.

Anatomy of an Illness by Norman Cousins.

You Can Knock Out AIDS With Vitamin C by Dr. Ian Brighthope.

Vitamin C as a Fundamental Medicine by Dr. London H. Smith.

Fight Fatigue by Dr. Ian Brighthope.

You Can Conquer Cancer by Ian Gawler.

Love, Medicine, and Miracles by Dr. Bernie Siegel.

Love, Peace, and Healing by Dr. Bernie Siegel.

Getting Well Again by O. Carl Simonton, Stephanie Matthews-Simonton, and James Creighton. J.P. Tarcher, 1978.

You Can Heal Your Life by Louise Hay.

Costs

Initial consultation (which is usually long): $80. Ten-day course: $240 for vitamin C, plus a $30 consulting fee. Follow-up vitamin C treatment: $23.50 per week for a 30 gram dose, plus a $30 consulting fee. Cost of weekend retreat and other services not submitted for publication. (All costs given in Australian dollars.)

Method of Payment

Payment for retreats must be made in advance. Payment for consultation must be made on that day.

The Gawler Foundation

Yarra Valley Living Centre
Rayner Court
Yarra Junction 3797
Australia

011-03-59-671730
Fax: 011-03-59-671715

Contact Person

Marion Wasley, Sheila Goodwin, Jan Akeroyd.

Primary Personnel

Dr. Ian Gawler, O.A.M., B.V.Sc.; Bob Sharples, Couns. Psych., MAPS.

Directions

One-and-a-half hour drive east of Melbourne.

Background

All programs are based on the experiences of Ian and Grace Gawler during Ian's recovery from a supposedly terminal bone cancer in 1975. They have worked with more than 10,000 patients since the programs began in 1981. They built on the results of that work and started the Gawler Foundation, which is a nonprofit, nondenominational association of cancer patients, their families, and concerned individuals. Its goals are: to provide active support for cancer patients and their families, with the aim of improving quality and quantity of life; to give recognition to the importance of the patient's contribution to the outcome of the treatment; to encourage patients to play an active, positive role in getting well again; to focus on the significance of nutrition, stress, positive thinking, meditation, and self-help groups; to foster research into the significance of the patient's role in cancer; to provide access to educational facilities and to sponsor relevant lectures, seminars, and workshops; to facilitate access to ancillary services such as dietitians, counselors, masseurs, etc., as an adjunct to medical treatments; to encourage communication and cooperation between patients and medical personnel; to provide assistance to disadvantaged patients where appropriate; to encourage and sponsor the establishment of affiliated self-help groups; and to take an active role in disseminating to the public information regarding cancer prevention.

Illness Addressed

All types of cancer.

Type of Program Offered

A ten-day residential program that creates an opportunity to review your life situation, seek clarity about your future direction, find meaning and purpose in your life, learn and practice self-help techniques, and experience meditation. There is also a twelve-week support group designed for cancer patients, their families, and their friends.

Related Readings

You Can Conquer Cancer by Ian Gawler.

Peace of Mind by Ian Gawler.

Women of Silence by Grace Gawler.

Inspiring People edited by Ian Gawler.

Length of Program/Stay

Ten-day residential program. Twelve-week support group for two-and-a-half hours each week.

Costs

Residential program: $1,870 for ten days. Support group: $180 for twelve-week series.

Method of Payment

Cash, checks, Visa, MasterCard, and Bankcard are all accepted.

The Hale Clinic

7 Park Crescent
London W1N 3HE
England

011-71-631-0156
011-71-637-3377
Fax: 011-71-323-1693

Primary Personnel

Teresa Hale, managing director.

Directions

The clinic is located on four floors in the prestigious Nash Terrace, only a few minutes from underground stations at Great Portland Street and Regents Park. Each floor is served by elevator for easy access by disabled visitors.

Background

The Hale Clinic was established in 1987. Its aim is to combine and integrate the principles of conventional and complementary medicine, as no one system of medicine has the whole answer to every medical problem. Great emphasis is placed on preventative medicine as a way of maintaining good health following treatment. Complementary medicine provides another dimension to what we think of as conventional medicine. While modern Western medicine tends to focus on treating specific illnesses and their symptoms, complementary medicine considers factors such as a patient's diet, temperament, work environment, and sleeping habits, among others, when prescribing treatment. There are 100 practitioners based at the Hale Clinic, twenty of whom are medical doctors, many of whom are multi-disciplinary. Although they differ considerably in the way they treat illness, they all view the practice of complementary medicine as helping the individual organism achieve its natural harmony and balance, thereby making it much less susceptible to illness and disease.

Illness Addressed

The Hale Clinic has pioneered research into chronic fatigue syndrome, multiple sclerosis, autism, cerebral palsy, and repetitive strain injury. A wide range of other illnesses are also addressed.

Type of Program Offered

Full range of complementary treatments, including acupuncture, Chinese herbal medicine, homeopathy, various types of massages and physical therapy, nutritional counseling, and many others.

Length of Program/Stay

Nonresidential.

Costs

Per practitioner.

Method of Payment

Cash and checks are accepted.

Hippocrates Health Centre of Australia

Elaine Avenue
Mudgeeraba 4213
Gold Coast
Queensland
Australia

011-07-5530-2860
Fax: 011-07-5530-3700

Primary Personnel

Ronald Bradley, B.A., M.A., founding director.

Directions

Fly to Coolangatta or bus to Burleigh Heads. The centre is a fifteen-minute taxi ride from either place or a one-hour drive south of Brisbane.

Background

Hippocrates, the founder of medicine, long ago demonstrated that wholesome natural foods can restore and maintain vibrant health. The body cleans and regenerates itself. If you have the proper nutrients, you can enjoy a life free from illness and pain. The Hippocrates self-help program focuses on nutritional, physical, mental, and emotional balance and harmony. Hippocrates Health Centre offers a complete health education, featuring Dr. Ann Wigmore's wheatgrass and living foods program, which, since 1960, has helped hundreds of thousands of people see that ideal health is natural for all of us. The program fosters regeneration, revitalization, and rejuvenation, leading to health, vigor, longevity, and youthful slimness.

Illness Addressed

Most health problems, including cancer, smoking, too much weight, and too much stress. However, students with contagious diseases may not attend.

Type of Program Offered

Dr. Wigmore's program offers a diet of 100 percent raw foods: sprouts, greens, fruits, vegetables, nuts, seeds, wheatgrass, and juices. It excludes all bread, flesh, dairy products, processed foods, and cooked foods. The curriculum features classes in gentle stretching exercises, wheatgrass, massage, meditation, self-improvement, positive thinking, breathing, food combining, menu planning, weight loss, sprouting, dehydrating foods, goals and affirmations, relaxation, stress reduction, visualization, kitchen equipment, and permaculture. The centre's recreational facilities include a heated pool and spa, a tennis court, a steam room, bushwalking, rebounding, ping-pong, and trampolining.

Related Readings

The Hippocrates Diet and Health Program by Dr. Ann Wigmore.

The Health Revolution by Ross Horne.

Improving on Pritikin by Ross Horne.

How I Conquered Cancer Naturally by Eydie Mae Hunsberger.

Length of Program/Stay

Minimum attendance is one week. Attendance of at least three weeks is strongly recommended.

Costs

One week: $795; two weeks: $1,495; three weeks: $2,195; four weeks: $2,895; five weeks: $3,595; six weeks: $4,295. If sufficient space is available, you may have your own private, comfortable motel-style room. If sufficient space is not available, or if you prefer to share, you may share with a partner, or with one other person of your sex. Tuition fees include all meals, room, learning and recreational activities, personal counseling with Hippocrates faculty, individual private health assessment (including iris analysis), textbook, and diploma. Massage and a wide variety of other personal health services are also available at additional cost.

Method of Payment

A deposit of half the tuition must be made in advance; the balance is paid upon arrival. Three credit cards are accepted: Bankcard, MasterCard, and Visa.

Hotaka Yojoen Holistic Health Center

7258-20 Ariake Hotaka-Cho
Minamiazumi-Gun
Nagano Prefecture 399-83
Japan

011-0263-83-5260
Fax: 011-0263-83-6670

Contact Person

Tamami Fukuda.

Primary Personnel

Shunsaku Fukuda, founder.

Directions

From Shinjuku station, take the Chuo line to Matsumoto. Transfer to the Oito line at Matsumoto, and get off at Hotaka or Ariake. There are also trains directly to Hotaka, such as the Azusa limited express on the Chuo line. The center is a ten-minute ride from Ariake or Hotaka. It is a three-hour train ride from Tokyo.

Background

This holistic health center is nestled on the slopes of the Japan Alps. The town of Hotaka is a rustic setting of hot springs, farms, pine trees, and honeysuckle. The center is nine years old and has ten tatami and Western-style accommodations.

Illness Addressed

Chronic diseases, including cancer.

Type of Program Offered

Macrobiotic natural whole foods diet, Onsen therapies (hand and foot germanium baths), natural hot spring baths, acupuncture, moxibustion, Shin integration (which is a bodywork like Rolfing), and shiatsu massage. On occasion, there are musical concerts, workshops on healing, and classes in ceramics, painting, and drawing. The center offers private health consultations, as well.

Length of Program/Stay

One-week stay is recommended, but a weekend is adequate if one has no other option.

Costs

Depends on length of stay. Up to seven nights: 8,500 yen per night (includes two meals and use of Onsen). From eight to twenty nights: 8,000 yen per night. Long-term stay (more than twenty nights): 7,500 yen per night during summer season (April 16 to October 14), 9,300 yen per night during winter season (October 15 to April 15). Initial acupuncture treatment with germanium bath treatment: 4,000 yen. Outpatient germanium bath treatment: 1,700 yen.

Method of Payment

Cash only is accepted.

Medical Research Inc.

Marlborough Cancer Help at Severne Natural Health Centre
Severne Street
Springlands
Blenheim
South Island
New Zealand

011-03-578-7335

Contact Person

Joy Breayley; Julia Davidson; Dale Yeoman.

Primary Personnel

Joy Breayley; Julia Davidson; Dale Yeoman.

Directions

Off Middle Renwick Road (the main highway to Nelson), look on the right at the second street past Springlands supermarket. The clinic is clearly signposted at the gates.

Background

Joy Breayley teaches meditation; Julia Davidson is a medical herbalist and nutritional counselor; Dale Yeoman conducts massage, teaching, and counseling. Together, they provide a holistic cancer treatment in conjunction with the patient's doctors. Medical Research is not a residential facility, but there are private accommodations close by.

Illness Addressed

Cancer.

Type of Program Offered

Herbal medicine, diet, lifestyle changes, enzymes, meditation, family counseling, visualization, relaxation, gentle massage, art therapy classes, group sessions, and herb teas served in the garden. Plus medical approach with Stephen Vallance, oncology nurse.

Costs

Costs not submitted for publication.

SUPPORT PROGRAMS

North America (Canada, United States)

Jan Abruzzo

17 Eighth Avenue
New York, New York 10014
United States

(212) 924-3924

Primary Personnel

Jan Abruzzo, C.S.W, psychotherapist, yoga therapist.

Directions

West Village. By appointment only.

Background

Ms. Abruzzo has been working with people with life-challenging illnesses for twenty years. For the past ten years, she has been in private practice, in consultation with Dr. Lawrence LeShan, Ph.D. She has advanced training as a psychotherapist, received her M.S.W. degree from Columbia University, and her B.S. from Cornell University. She is also a therapeutic yoga and meditation teacher, certified by Integral Yoga Institute. She is a founding member of the Commonweal Cancer Help Program, and continues to participate in Commonweal's annual Symington Foundation invitational conference on new directions in cancer care. She has trained with Dr. Dean Ornish's Program for Reversing Heart Diseases, and is doing this work within her private practice. She has worked extensively, but not exclusively, with people with medical challenges. Her practice includes people confronted with nonmedical problems as well.

Illness Addressed

Cancer, heart disease, amyotrophic lateral sclerosis (Lou Gehrig's disease), and any other medical illness, as well as nonmedical challenges.

Type of Service Provided

Psychotherapy, yoga therapy, and stress management, for individuals and couples.

Related Readings

Cancer as a Turning Point by Lawrence LeShan, Ph.D. Plume Books, 1994.

Length of Program/Stay

Determined by client's need.

Costs

$100 per session. Sliding scale available.

Method of Payment

Checks or cash is accepted. Reimbursable by most insurance, depending on individual's policy.

AeroStat Air & Land Ambulance, Inc.

8690 Aero Drive, #142
San Diego, California 92123
United States

(619) 573-0189
011-52-66-300080 (Mexico)

Contact Person

Julayne Smithson, R.N., chief flight nurse; Shane Smithson, chief pilot.

Background

AeroStat Air & Land Ambulance, Inc., is a United States corporation based in San Diego, California. It has been in business for six years. AeroStat de Mexico is a Mexican corporation offering ground and air ambulance services within Mexico. Both companies primarily service the cancer clinics in Mexico. The Mexican corporation is based in Playas de Tijuana, Mexico, and offers United States-equipped ambulances and United States nurses on site in Mexico.

Illness Addressed

These corporations specialize in the transport of cancer patients or patients seeking any kind of alternative treatment.

Type of Service Provided

Air ambulance, ground ambulance, and escort service worldwide to any of the cancer clinics in Mexico. This escort service is used for patients who need assistance in getting to Mexico, but who do not need air ambulance. It has technicians and nurses who go along with patients on commercial flights, and can even place a certified FAA bed on a commercial airliner. Due to many years of reliable service, it holds exclusive contracts with many of the facilities in Playas and in Tijuana.

Costs

Varies depending on the individual case, the distance to be transported, and other factors.

Method of Payment

Personal checks, cashier's checks, credit cards, and payment options are accepted.

The American Health Institute, Inc.

12381 Wilshire Boulevard
Los Angeles, California 90025
United States

(310) 207-3144
Fax: (310) 207-3342
Internet: http://www.ahealth.com/ahi/

Contact Person

Janet Hranicky, Ph.D.

Primary Personnel

Janet Hranicky, Ph.D.

Directions

405 Freeway (San Diego Freeway) to Wilshire Boulevard West. Continue on Wilshire Boulevard for two miles.

Background

Janet Hranicky, Ph.D., the founder of the American Health Institute, Inc., is one of the few experts in the world to provide a solid theoretical foundation for the definition of stress and to demonstrate its link to emotional patterns and cancer. Her program is the result of more than eighteen years of education, research, and clinical experience in the field of psychoneuroimmunology and cancer, during which time she has personally worked with thousands of cancer patients. Dr. Hranicky trained extensively with Carl Simonton, M.D. She was his associate at the Simonton Cancer Center for over fifteen years, where she helped to conduct a National New Patient Program. She has trained professionals across the United States, and has lectured throughout the United States and Europe. Dr. Hranicky and Dr. Simonton are designing the world's first systematized intervention and training model for the field of psychoneuroimmunology to provide quality standards for mind-body medicine. This model will be made available to hospitals and medical systems throughout the world.

Illness Addressed

The mental/emotional/stress-related aspects of cancer.

Treatment Offered

This is a self-contained interactive treatment program to address the mind-body and cancer. The program has been designed to empower individuals with cancer to sucessfully maximize their recovery potential, and it is ideal for use in conjunction with standard medical treatment. The program consists of: two interactive videotapes covering the ten components of the Hranicky Program (three hours); training workbook, *The Hranicky Mind Body Cancer Program,* covering the components of the program in more depth and detail; ten audio tapes; and the Kohler computerized stress profile, adapted clinically for the psychosocial treatment of cancer by Dr. Janet Hranicky.

Length of Treatment/Stay

Variable.

Costs

Total cost for the interactive audio-video program, training workbook, and stress profile for cancer is $295 plus tax, shipping, and handling. To order, call: (800) 392-2623, or fax: (310) 207-3342.

Method of Payment

Personal, cashier's, and traveler's checks; and Visa and MasterCard are accepted.

Ruth Bolletino, Ph.D.

441 West End Avenue, #1B
New York, New York 10024
United States

(212) 496-9136

315 Sixth Avenue
Brooklyn, New York 11215
United States

(718) 768-7953

Primary Personnel

Ruth Bolletino, Ph.D.

Background

Dr. Bolletino, a clinical psychologist, is trained in a wide variety of approaches to the human condition, and has had wide experience working with people with catastrophic illness.

Illness Addressed

Primarily cancer; also HIV and AIDS.

Type of Service Provided

Dr. Bolletino sees people with cancer, HIV, and AIDS for psychotherapy aimed at mobilizing the client's self-healing abilities. She also offers counseling to family members of clients. Also, with Dr. Lawrence LeShan, Dr. Bolletino works with individual cancer patients using a "marathon" model of brief, intensive psychotherapy. A typical marathon is held for five or six days, each involving two to five hours of psychotherapeutic work. The first session is usually held with Dr. LeShan, followed by days of intensive work with Dr. Bolletino. The concluding hour is held with both therapists.

Related Readings

Cancer as a Turning Point by Lawrence LeShan, Revised edition. Plume Books, 1994.

Method of Payment

Cash and checks are accepted.

The Bresler Center, Inc.

115 South Topanga Canyon Boulevard, #198
Topanga, California 90290
United States

(800) 95-RELAX

Contact Person

Dr. David Bresler.

Background

Dr. Bresler has been leading support groups for people with chronic pain, cancer, and other catastrophic illnesses, for over twenty-five years.

Illness Addressed

Chronic pain, cancer, heart disease, diabetes, asthma, degenerative neurological diseases, and other catastrophic illnesses.

Type of Service Provided

Psychotherapy, relaxation training, acupuncture, visualization, guided imagery, stress management, nutritional counseling, homeopathy, self-help, support, and study groups.

Related Readings

Free Yourself From Pain by Dr. Bresler. Simon and Schuster, 1979; Fireside, 1984; Alphabooks, 1996.

Length of Program/Stay

Five to seven days for healing retreats in Hawaii. Once weekly for Los Angeles groups.

Costs

Variable.

Method of Payment

Cash, checks, Visa, and MasterCard are accepted. The center does not accept insurance.

Burzynski Patients Organization

P.O. Box 1770
Pacific Palisades, California 90272
United States

Contact Persons

Mariann and Jack Kunnari, (218) 638-2408; Alice Cedillo, (214) 321-9334; Ed Reynolds, (718) 409-6857; Robin Ressel, (417) 886-6145.

Background

This organization was formed to provide information to patients who are considering being treated by Dr. Stanislaw Burzynski, as well as to current patients of Dr. Burzynski. It also raises money to help pay for the legal defense of Dr. Burzynski through the Burzynski Legal Defense Fund.

Illness Addressed

Cancer, including brain tumors, non-Hodgkins lymphoma, prostate, breast, and others. Autoimmune diseases, including lupus, multiple sclerosis, rheumatoid arthritis, HIV, and others.

Type of Information Offered

The organization has a Patient-to-Patient line, (415) 750-3035, to provide prospective and current Burzynski cancer patients with the names and phone numbers of current and former patients who have been helped by the Burzynski treatment and who have the same type of cancer. The Hotline number for updates regarding Dr. Burzynski, the Burzynski Clinic, and the patient organization is (317) 971-6536.

Related Readings

Reclaiming Our Health by John Robbins.
Options by Richard Walters.
The Cancer Industry by Ralph Moss, Ph.D.
Questioning Chemotherapy by Ralph Moss, Ph.D.
Alternative Medicine by Burton Goldberg Group.

Costs

For information about Dr. Burzynski and the history of antineoplastons, the cost is $25. For the same information and a videotape about Dr. Burzynski, his patients, and their struggle for freedom of medical choice, please send $50. Make checks payable to Burzynski Legal Defense Fund.

Cancer Counseling Center

1515 Lake Martin Drive
Kent, Ohio 44240
United States

(216) 922-1855
(216) 626-3115

7 Hidden Hollow
Pittsford, New York 14534
United States

(716) 833-1183

Contact Person

Receptionist.

Primary Personnel

David G. Zimpfer, Ed.D., L.P.C.C., N.C.C.

Directions

Located in a residential area just off State Route 43, about four miles north of Kent. Easy access from Cleveland and Akron airports and from Ohio Turnpike.

Background

Treatment includes methods of Dr. Carl Simonton, Dr. Bernie Siegel, and the Voluntary Controls Program at Menninger Clinic. It is based on the assumption that illness can be overcome and that the person can exert some control over the healing process. Illness may come to be seen as an opportunity for change or fulfillment. Quality of life is emphasized. Bed-and-breakfast facilities on site are offered at nominal cost for persons who do not live in the area. Maps and lists of local motels and restaurants can also be supplied. Treatment is seen as complementary to any medical care being provided.

Illness Addressed

Cancer and other autoimmune diseases (e.g., rheumatoid arthritis, multiple sclerosis, lupus erythematosus, Sjogren's disease, Hashimoto's disease). Also other illnesses or physical disabilities in which quality of life is affected or which cause much anxiety.

Type of Service Provided

Biofeedback, guided imagery, psychosynthesis, meditation, relaxation and breathing, hypnosis, dreamwork, art therapy, and other methods are used as needed to promote optimal personal control and enhance immune functioning. Stress, pain, loneliness, helplessness, fatigue, and fatalism are dealt with. Counseling includes discussion of: the will to recover, death and dying, secondary gains of illness, stress factors, becoming an informed and assertive patient, taking responsibility for one's health, emotional issues that may aggravate the disease process, spirituality, resolution of interpersonal problems, love, and forgiveness. Exercise, nutrition, and continuation of personal productivity are also emphasized. Treatment is highly individualized and is conducted on a one-to-one basis. It is very helpful for a patient to have a partner, close friend, or loved one as a supporter. Such a person will be asked to attend at least some sessions. Several times a year an intensive group therapy program is offered. Essentially the same treatment is provided as in individual therapy. The group program is especially useful for those who travel a long distance, for those who wish to reduce costs, and for those who desire the close interpersonal support that develops in a group. Support persons are encouraged to enroll and participate along with the client.

Related Readings

Cancer as a Turning Point by Lawrence LeShan. Plume Books, 1994.

Minding the Body, Mending the Mind by Joan Borysenko. Addison-Wesley, 1987.

Peace, Love, and Healing by Bernie Siegel. Harper & Row, 1989.

Healing Words by Larry Dossey. HarperCollins, 1993.

The Psychology of Mind-Body Healing by Ernest Rossi. W.W. Norton, 1993.

Imagery for Getting Well by Deidre Brigham. W.W. Norton, 1994.

Books, audio tapes, and nutritional supplements are available through mail order. Catalog supplied upon request.

Length of Program/Stay

Clients who commute will generally have a two-hour session once or twice a week, depending on their level of anxiety and physical stamina. Treatment is arranged on a more frequent and intensive basis (several visits over two or three days or a full week) for those who come from a greater distance. Home and hospital visits can be arranged for people unable to travel. Individual treatment most commonly extends for twenty-five to thirty hours. Upon evaluation, a decision is made whether to extend, to go on a reduced schedule of "booster" sessions, or to terminate. Group therapy extends for a full-time week of five days.

Costs

$90 per hour of individual counseling. No additional fee for persons who accompany the client to individual counseling. Group therapy $995 per week. Reduced rate for support persons in group therapy.

Method of Payment

Cash, personal checks, and money orders are accepted. Most health insurance contracts cover at least some costs. Insurance claims can be filed on the client's behalf. In some cases, the insurance carrier can be billed directly for its contribution. Payment for individual treatment is due upon completion of each session. Monthly billing is possible after financial responsibility has been established. Group therapy requires a $100 advance deposit to reserve a place; the balance is due at the start of the program. Extended payment programs can sometimes be arranged.

Cancer Counselling Center

P.O. Box 711
Station "A"
Toronto, Ontario M5W 1G2
Canada

(416) 778-4567

Primary Personnel

Dr. M. Cole Cohen, Ph.D., clinical director; Tucker I. Feller, M.A., M.Ed., program research.

Background

The program has evolved from the now generally-accepted principle that beliefs, feelings, attitudes, and lifestyle integrally affect our health. The center regularly updates its program to integrate recent findings on the theory and practice of psycho-social factors that influence the reinstatement and maintenance of health, including: social support, visualization, personal relationships, diet, physical activity, informed decisions, and stress management. The center uses these lifestyle choices as vehicles to help clients in their medical recovery and emotional health.

Illness Treated

Although most clients are individuals with cancer and their families, the techniques and principles involved are also sought out by persons with conditions such as allergies, asthma, and arthritis.

Treatment Offered

Counselling for individuals, families, and groups based on the Simonton method of integrating mind and body in the healing process. Individual and family counselling, including: how to deal with the effects of cancer on family and friends; ways of being proactive in the treatment of one's medical condition; how to participate in one's own wellness program; how to replace a stress response with a relaxation response; and how to create individualized visualizations.

The center also offers a five-day, in-depth group program based on the work of Dr. O. Carl Simonton and others in the field of psychosocial oncology. Participants learn techniques to promote their health through lifestyle analysis, individual counselling, emotional awareness, education in immunosuppressant factors, and visualization coaching. Key program components include: links between stress and illness; individualized visualization clinic; group and individual counselling; techniques for enhanced immune function; the influence of emotions, attitudes, and beliefs on health; coping with the fears of death and recurrence of illness; and overcoming obstacles to recovery.

The center provides a reference service for clients who wish to further educate themselves in the scientific literature regarding mind-body interaction, psychoneuroimmunology, visualization, and the function of hormones and neuropeptides. Clients have access to studies that ground the theory and practice underlying the demonstrations, practice, and didactic sessions found in the program.

Related Readings

Achterberg, J. *Imagery in Healing.* Boston: New Science Library.

Borysenko, J. *Minding the Body, Mending the Mind.* Reading, Massachusetts: Addison-Wesley, 1987.

Cousins, N. *Anatomy of an Illness.* New York: W.W. Norton, 1979.

Green, R. and Green, M. "Relaxation increases salivary immunoglobulin A." *Psychological Reports,* 1987, 61:623-629.

Greer, S. "Cancer and the mind." *British Journal of Psychiatry,* 1983, 143: 535-543.

LeShan, L. *Cancer as a Turning Point.* New York: E.P. Dutton, 1989.

Rider, M. and Achterberg, J. "Effect of music-assisted imagery on neutrophils and lymphocytes." *Biofeedback and Self-Regulation,* 1989, 14 (3): 247-257.

Siegel, B. *Love, Medicine, and Miracles.* New York: Harper and Row, 1986.

Simonton, O.C., Simonton, S. and Creighton, J.L. *Getting Well Again.* Los Angeles: J.P. Tarcher, 1978.

Spiegel, D. et al. "Effect of psychosocial treatment on survival of patients with metastatic breast cancer." *Lancet,* 1989, October 14: 888-891.

Spiegel, D., and Bloom, J. "Group therapy and hypnosis reduce metastatic breast cancer carcinoma pain." *Psychosomatic Medicine,* 1983, 45 (4): 333-339.

Length of Treatment

Five-day group program. Follow-up sessions as scheduled with client.

Costs

There is a sliding fee schedule for the five-day group program. There is no charge for a spouse/support person. Full tuition is $1,500. The center has not refused anyone on the grounds of an inability to pay. Individual counselling: $90/hour. Individual version of group program: $75/hour.

Method of Payment

Several forms of group insurance cover all or part of the program. Participants are encouraged to check with their own agent or the benefit personnel at their company to determine if their insurance or group health benefit policy covers such treatment. The center will gladly complete insurance forms provided.

Cancer Support and Education Center

1035 Pine Street
Menlo Park, California 94025
United States

(415) 327-6166
Fax: (415) 327-2018

Contact Person

Peggy Rogers, director of client services.

Primary Personnel

William Collinge, Ph.D., clinical supervisor; Karen Haas, M.A., director; Peggy Rogers, director of client services.

Directions

Take Highway 101 north or south, exit at Marsh Road/Atherton. You will be on Marsh Road, heading west. Turn left onto Middlefield, then right onto Oak Grove Avenue. Turn right onto Pine Street. The center is located between El Camino and Middlefield, and between Oak Grove Avenue and Ravenswood Avenue.

Background

Illness can serve as an opportunity to heal emotionally, physically, and spiritually, for both the patient and for family members. Within a safe environment, patients can "use the illness as a teacher" to learn about who they are, what is meaningful in life, and how they can develop deep intimate relationships with others.

Illness Addressed

People with cancer and their families make up the largest number of clients, but anyone with any kind of illness or issue is welcome.

Type of Service Provided

The center provides four types of programs:

1. A self-empowerment program for people with illness—a structured, in-depth, mind/body program that meets once a week for ten weeks, or every day for two weeks (sixty hours).

2. Individual, couples, family therapy, using a variety of modalities (cognitive, somatic, art therapy, play therapy for children).

3. Kids Helping Kids—a support group for children who have an ill parent or relative.

Meets weekly for eight sessions—children are encouraged to repeat the group as long as needed. KHK includes meetings for parents to learn how to help their children.

4. Intern/Training programs for students and professionals.

Related Readings

Cancer as a Turning Point by Lawrence LeShan.
Love, Medicine, and Miracles by Bernie Siegel.
Full Catastrophe Living by John Kabat-Zinn.
Getting Well Again by Carl and Stephanie Simonton.
Don't Go Away Mad by James Creighton.
Getting the Love You Want by Harville Hendricks.
The Human Patient by Rachel Naomi Remen.
How to Help Children Through a Parent's Serious Illness.

Length of Program/Stay

Varies greatly, although the average patient attends the sixty-hour program once or twice.

Costs

Self-empowerment program: $1,600 for two persons (client with illness and a significant other or support person). Private sessions: $75/hour. Kids Helping Kids: free. Intern/Training Program: $2,600 for one year. Reimbursable by insurance and sliding scale, including scholarships.

Method of Payment

Cash, checks, Visa, MasterCard, and payment plans are accepted. Insurance is accepted from anyone with an illness who has psychological service coverage.

Cancer Support Community

185 Lundys Lane
San Francisco, California 94110
United States

(415) 648-9400

Contact Person

Debra Ballinger, executive director; Patrick Thornton, Ph.D., clinical director.

Directions

This center is in the Bernal Heights area of San Francisco.

Background

This is a nonprofit organization founded in 1986 by two women with cancer who, out of their own experience, created a community to meet the needs of people with cancer, their families, and their friends. The entire staff has had experience with cancer.

Illness Addressed

Cancer.

Type of Service Provided

Cancer Support Community offers understanding, support, and guidance to people with cancer and those who care about them. Its programs address the physical, mental, emotional, and spiritual needs of participants. Services include a variety of support groups for people with cancer, their families, and their friends; education programs (such as training and imagery, stress reduction, nutrition, and pain management); individual, couple, and family counseling; grief support; and library and referral services. Social activities (such as community parties and picnics) and volunteer opportunities occur regularly. Support groups are also offered in Cantonese and Spanish.

Costs

All programs are free. Donations are accepted.

Center for Attitudinal Healing

33 Buchanan Drive
Sausalito, California 94965
United States

(415) 331-6161

Primary Personnel

Don Goewey, executive director; Louise Franklin, fund development; Cristina Chanteloup, administration; Malinda Luger, finance; Valerie Henderson, adult program; Jimmy Pete, children and youth program; Jennifer Andrews, volunteers; Marilyn Robinson, education.

Background

The center was started in 1975 by Dr. Gerald Jampolsky and five volunteers, working with children with cancer. The philosophy of attitudinal healing maintains that it is not people, places, or things outside ourselves that cause us to be unhappy, but our response to these things. Love is the most powerful healing force in the world. The focus of the center is to provide emotional and spiritual support to people in a support-group setting. Education and presentations are done locally and around the world. Attitudinal healing principles are a distillation of universal truths that transcend cultural and language lines.

Illness Addressed

All forms of cancer, heart disease, HIV, and AIDS.

Type of Service Provided

Emotional and spiritual support groups that utilize the principles of attitudinal healing.

Related Readings

Love Is Letting Go of Fear by Gerald G. Jampolsky, M.D.

Teach Only Love by Gerald G. Jampolsky, M.D.

Out of Darkness Into the Light by Gerald G. Jampolsky, M.D.

Love Is the Answer by Gerald G. Jampolsky, M.D., and Diane Cirincione.

Who Dies, Embracing the Beloved by Stephen Levine.

To See Differently by Susan Trout

Trust the Force by Dr. Todd Davidson.

Love, Medicine, and Miracles by Bernie Siegel.

Length of Program/Stay

The groups are open and ongoing.

Costs

There is no charge for support group services. Workshops are offered four times per year; prices vary.

Colorado Outward Bound School

945 Pennsylvania Avenue
Denver, Colorado 80203
United States

(800) 477-2627 ext. 6974

Contact Person

Sian Haurer.

Directions

The courses are run out of Leadville, Colorado. Directions will be sent to participants when they enter the program.

Background

Started in 1961, Colorado Outward Bound is the nation's oldest wilderness adventure school. It promotes education, service, and personal growth through wilderness experience. While not a "survival" school in the literal sense, Outward Bound provides participants with the tools needed for success in the outdoors. Outward Bound is offering a course specifically designed to allow women who are surviving cancer the opportunity to come together, to share the struggle, and to work together to overcome the challenge of cancer. The activities of the course act as a mirror, providing valuable lessons that apply to surviving cancer and living life to its fullest.

Illness Addressed

Survivors of cancer.

Type of Service Provided

The course provides opportunities to explore methods of coping with challenge, overcome seemingly impossible tasks, draw upon the strength and ideas of oneself and others, and explore fear, passion, friendship, and a sense of community. A sample itinerary includes: problem-solving initiatives and trust-building activities, rock climbing and rappelling, peak climb, ropes course, and time for personal reflection.

Length of Program/Stay

Three to five days.

Costs

$130 per person per day, plus $75 application fee. Includes all instruction, specialized camping and safety equipment, secondary accident insurance, transportation while on course, and food.

Method of Payment

Cash, checks, Visa, and MasterCard are accepted. Scholarships are available.

Commonweal Cancer Help Program

P.O. Box 316
Bolinas, California 94924
United States

(415) 868-0970

Contact Person

Waz Thomas, program coordinator.

Primary Personnel

Michael Lerner, Ph.D., president; Rachel Naomi Remen, M.D., medical director; Virginia Veach, Ph.D., M.F.C.C.

Directions

Please call first. From the Golden Gate Bridge, go approximately two-and-a-half miles to Stinson Beach/Highway 1 exit. Continue about ten miles to Stinson Beach. Go five miles past town of Stinson Beach, take the first road to the left, just past the end of the lagoon. Make a left again at the end of this short connecting road and go about one mile. Turn left at the stop sign. Go half a mile, turn right on Mesa Road. Go approximately two-and-a-quarter miles, enter driveway on left.

Background

Weeklong workshops take place approximately bimonthly, at the sixty-acre Commonweal site in the Point Reyes National Seashore north of San Francisco. The program was the subject of an hour-long documentary by Bill Moyers, "Wounded Heavens," part of his award-winning PBS documentary *Healing and the Mind*.

Illness Addressed

Cancer.

Type of Service Provided

Commonweal Cancer Help Program is an educational program, not a cancer therapy. It is designed to help participants reduce the stress of cancer, explore better health habits, be with others facing the same difficulties, and consider information on both established and complementary therapeutic options. The daily program includes support groups led by a trained psychologist, yoga and meditation, deep relaxation and imagery, massage therapy, work with sand trays, and healthy vegetarian meals. Participants must be under the care of an oncologist or other allopathic physician.

Related Readings

Choices in Healing: Integrating the Best of Conventional and Complementary Approaches to Cancer by Michael Lerner. MIT Press, 1994.

Length of Program/Stay

One week.

Costs

$1,480. Same fee for family member or other support person. Some scholarship support is available.

Method of Payment

Checks, MasterCard, and Visa are accepted.

Consciousness Research and Training Project Inc.

315 East 68th Street, Box 9G
New York, New York 10021
United States

Primary Personnel

Joyce Goodrich, Ph.D., project director.

Background

This is a nonprofit training and research project based on Dr. Lawrence LeShan's research and practice in meditation and healing. The project's work has been ongoing for over twenty-five years.

Illness Addressed

Cancer and others, although illnesses are not addressed per se. Rather, the project establishes an environment in which the process of self-healing can take place as an adjunct to medical treatment.

Type of Service Provided

Five-day retreats and seminars are held around the country to train people to use the method. Occasionally, the project sends out a newsletter to those who have been trained. Applications and schedules for the training are available upon request.

Length of Program/Stay

Five full days, residential for Introductory Seminar. Three to four full days for optional Advanced Seminars.

Costs

$275 tuition for the five days. Room and board costs about $250.

Method of Payment

Checks and cash are accepted.

Exceptional Cancer Patients (ECaP)

300 Plaza Middlesex
Middletown, Connecticut 06457
United States

(860) 343-5950
Fax: (860) 343-5956

Contact Person

Tim Albaitis, director.

Background

Exceptional Cancer Patients, or ECaP, is a nonprofit organization founded by Bernie Siegel, M.D., to provide group support for cancer patients. It is used as an adjunctive therapy; patients are urged to participate in their healing process.

Illness Addressed

Cancer, AIDS/HIV, and other chronic or life-threatening illnesses.

Type of Service Provided

Support groups, individual and family therapy workshops.

Related Readings

Love, Medicine, and Miracles by Bernie S. Siegel, M.D. Harper & Row, 1986.
Peace, Love, and Healing by Bernie S. Siegel, M.D. Harper & Row.
How to Live Between Office Visits by Bernie S. Siegel, M.D.

Costs

A sliding fee scale is available. Mail-order books, audio tapes, and videotapes are available. Free catalog sent upon request.

Method of Payment

Cash, checks, Visa, and MasterCard are accepted.

The Georgia CancerHelp Program

26 Briar Gate Lane
Marietta, Georgia 30066
United States

(770) 428-9228
Fax: (770) 429-0276

Center for New Beginnings
Dahlonega, Georgia 30533
United States

Contact Person

Colin Tipping or JoAnn Tipping, founder-directors.

Primary Personnel

Medical doctors, chiropractor, psychotherapist, minister, nutritionist, massage therapist, and a mind-body therapist.

Directions

From Atlanta, north on GA 400 to Dahlonega.

Background

The Georgia CancerHelp Program has been in operation since 1993, running five-day healing retreats that focus on emotional and spiritual healing as well as mental factors. Some educational material is given on alternative treatments. The program is operated under Together-We-Heal, Inc., a nonprofit organization.

Illness Addressed

Primarily cancer, but also multiple sclerosis, chronic fatigue syndrome, and HIV/AIDS.

Type of Service Provided

Retreats, workshops, and healing vacations, which include group counseling and support, art therapy, individual counseling, energy healing, bodywork and massage, forgiveness, relaxation, and information about holistic treatments.

Related Readings

Books by Michael Lerner, Rachael Naomi Remen, Bernie Siegel, Greg Anderson, Carolyn Myss, Lawrence LeShan, and Deepak Chopra.

Length of Program/Stay

Five or seven days. Also three-day weekend workshops.

Costs

Five-day retreat: $575 plus a donation. Bahamas healing vacations: $1,900 to $4,000. Weekend workshops: $225.

Method of Payment

Cash, checks, Visa, and MasterCard are accepted. Since chiropractic work is involved, if the patient is covered for chiropractic, some of the costs are recoverable from insurance.

Harmony Hill of Union

East 7362 Highway 106
Union, Washington 98592
United States

(360) 898-2363
Fax: (360) 898-2364

Contact Person

Gretchen Schodde, A.R.N.P., M.N., family nurse practitioner, executive director.

Primary Personnel

Joy Carey, Ph.D.; Chuck Buser, M.D.

Directions

From Seattle, take I-5 south to Tacoma, then Highway 106 West toward Bremerton. Highway 3 south toward Shelton/Beleair, Highway 106 toward Twanoh State Park/Union. Approximately thirteen miles on left, just before Alder Brook Inn.

Background

Harmony Hill cancer retreats were inspired by the Commonweal Cancer Help Program in Bolinas, California, and established in 1994. Participants learn ways to reduce the stress of cancer, provide mutual support, and learn health-promoting skills. The program's philosophy is to provide the opportunity for individuals living with cancer to regain a sense of meaning and well-being in their lives by moving beyond crisis.

Illness Addressed
Cancer, stress.

Type of Service Provided
Education and support for participants to develop tools for dealing with cancer. Therapies include qi gong, healing with music, group support sessions, sand tray, reiki energy balancing, and massage. Healthful meals and snacks are also provided.

Length of Program/Stay
Four-and-a-half days.

Costs
$750. Includes program, lodging, and meals.

Method of Payment
Cash, checks, and Visa are accepted. The program does not accept insurance at this time.

HOPE Cancer Health Society

2574 West Broadway, Suite 1
Vancouver, British Columbia V6K 2G2
Canada

(604) 732-3412

Contact Person
Moyra White, founder; Jean Rae.

Primary Personnel
All are cancer survivors.

Directions
Located in the Kitsilano area of Vancouver. Closest major intersection is MacDonald Street and West Broadway.

Background

The HOPE cancer program was founded in 1980 by Claude Dosdall and Moyra White. Both are cancer survivors. Since 1980, HOPE has helped thousands of cancer patients and their families deal with the crisis of cancer away from the hospital environment. It is an intensive, structured, self-help cancer recovery program. Through HOPE, patients learn to take an active part in their fight for recovery. HOPE believes that a partnership between the patient and the health professional is the only effective way to defeat cancer.

Illness Addressed

All kinds of cancer.

Type of Service Provided

The program teaches techniques for stress reduction, relaxation, exercise, nutrition, visualization, and communication. Ongoing individual and group support assists the patient and the family to deal effectively with the devastating physical and emotional effects of cancer and its treatments.

Related Readings

My God, I Thought You'd Died by Claude Dosdall and Joanne Broatch. Bantam-Seal Books, 1986.

Getting Well Again by O. Carl Simonton, M.D., Stephanie Matthews-Simonton, and James Creighton. J.P. Tarcher, 1978.

Length of Program/Stay

Workshops can run for one day, one evening, or a full weekend. Individual and family counseling can be ongoing.

Costs

Program costs vary from $50 to $395 (for retreats). Subsidies are usually available for those who need them.

Method of Payment

Cash and checks are accepted.

The Intimacy and Healing Project

P.O. Box 2002
Sebastopol, California 95472
United States

(800) 745-1837

Contact Person
William Collinge, Ph.D., director.

Primary Personnel
William Collinge, Ph.D.; Abigail Platt, NCPsyA.

Directions
Programs are in various locations. Call or write for schedule.

Background
This program is for couples involved in an intimate relationship in which one partner has a serious illness. The project includes workshops, retreats, and educational materials to help couples learn to use their intimate relationship to promote healing in the ill partner, and to enhance the quality of their lives together.

Illness Addressed
Cancer, chronic fatigue syndrome, fibromyalgia, HIV, heart disease, and other chronic or degenerative illnesses.

Type of Service Provided
Therapeutic and educational support for the patient and intimate other, focusing on their relationship: how illness affects the relationship, and how intimacy can be used as a stimulus to evoke healing responses in the patient. Retreats, workshops, video and audiotapes, and printed matter.

Related Readings
The American Holistic Health Association Complete Guide to Alternative Medicine by William Collinge. Warner Books, 1996.
Recovering from Chronic Fatigue Syndrome: A Guide to Self-Empowerment. Putnam, 1993.
The Book of Subtle Energy by William Collinge.

Length of Program/Stay
One-day workshops, weekend workshops and residential retreats, and week-long retreats.

Costs

Costs vary, depending on location and length of program.

Method of Payment

Cash, checks, Visa, and MasterCard are accepted. Patients pay full fees up front, and a statement is given to seek reimbursement from insurance company (as a group therapy/mental health service).

Lawrence LeShan, Ph.D.

263 West End Avenue
New York, New York 10023
United States

(212) 724-5802

Primary Personnel

Lawrence LeShan, Ph.D.

Background

Lawrence LeShan, an experimental psychologist, has spent four decades in research and psychotherapeutic work with cancer patients. He is generally considered a pioneer in dealing with emotional factors in the treatment of cancer.

Illness Addressed

Cancer.

Type of Service Provided

Dr. LeShan will see people for a single consultation to evaluate their total situation. If appropriate, he will refer them and/or their families to specialists in psychotherapy. Dr. LeShan, with his associate Dr. Ruth Bolletino, also works with individual cancer patients using a "marathon" model of brief intensive psychotherapy. A typical marathon is held for five or six days, each involving two to five hours of psychotherapeutic work. The first session is usually held with Dr. LeShan, followed by days of intensive work with Dr. Bolletino. The client meets with both therapists for the concluding session.

Related Readings

Cancer as a Turning Point by Lawrence LeShan. Plume Books, 1994.

Costs

Costs not submitted for publication but are based on a sliding scale.

Method of Payment

Cash and checks are accepted.

Mind/Body Center

845 Via de la Paz, Suite 7
Pacific Palisades, California 90272
United States

(310) 454-0920

Contact Person

Michelle Leclaire O'Neill, Ph.D., R.N.

Primary Personnel

Michelle Leclaire O'Neill, Ph.D., R.N.

Directions

Take the Santa Monica Freeway to Pacific Coast Highway. Take the Tenescal Canyon exit right, then go uphill to Sunset Boulevard. Turn right and go one block to the light at Via de la Paz. Turn right here; the building is on the right.

Background

Dr. O'Neill believes that cancer and other life-challenging illnesses can be construed as a signal for change. If one moves away from the hopelessness and fear that a life-challenging diagnosis often brings, and toward a belief that beneficial things are still possible, then the illness can alter the life of both the patient and his or her family in a constructive way. To move toward a true and lasting state of well-being, Dr. O'Neill addresses the desires and needs that well up from the unconscious, which manifests through our emotions and dreams. If we attend to our needs, then disease is an unwelcome visitor.

Illness Addressed

Cancer, HIV, and postpartum depression. This method is applicable to all diseases of the immune system.

Type of Service Provided

Twelve-week support groups for cancer patients and their families; one-day seminars; individual and family counseling; and home and hospital visits.

Related Readings

Getting Well Again by O. Carl Simonton, M.D., Stephanie Matthews-Simonton, and James Creighton. J.P. Tarcher, 1978.

Love, Medicine, and Miracles by Bernie Siegel, M.D.

Cassette tapes on healing, including *The Healer Within* by Michelle Leclaire O'Neill, are available through mail order.

Length of Program/Stay

Twelve-week group program; individual counseling, six to twelve weeks. These are outpatient programs.

Costs

$60 per week for group program. $120 per hour for private counseling. $150 for all-day sessions.

Method of Payment

Cash or checks are accepted. The center will help the patient fill out insurance forms for reimbursement.

O Ka Mana Ka Ho'ola

P.O. Box 1236
Kamuela, Hawaii 96743
United States

(808) 885-0995
(808) 885-6777
(808) 885-7547
Fax: (808) 885-4998

Contact Person

Noni Kuhns, program director.

Primary Personnel

Fran Woollard, R.N.; Nancy Bouvet, administrator; Suzanne Simonds, operations director.

Directions

Arrive Kona Airport, Big Island of Hawaii. Located on the Kohala coast, near Mauna Kea and Mauna Lani resorts, on the beach.

Background

This program is educational and is not a treatment. It does not advise participants on which therapies they should choose. All participants must be under the care of a primary physician or an oncologist, and be well enough to benefit from the program.

Illness Addressed

All types of cancer.

Type of Service Provided

A seven-day residential retreat aimed at reducing stress and providing an intensive experience of mutual support and intellectual and experiential learning, in a safe and nurturing environment.

Related Readings

This program is modeled directly on the Commonweal Cancer Help Program, located in Bolinas, California, directed by Michael Lerner, Ph.D. and Rachel Naomi Remen, M.D., and featured in the PBS-Bill Moyers documentary, *Healing and the Mind.*

Length of Program/Stay

Week-long workshop.

Costs

$1,000. The cost is the same for family member or support person.

Method of Payment

Checks or cash is accepted.

Psychosomatics

1729 Collingwood Drive
San Diego, California 92109
United States

(619) 272-9869
(619) 461-9527

Primary Personnel

Dr. Robert Price.

Directions

Central San Diego, near the airport.

Background

Dr. Price has been working professionally in psychoneuroimmunology, also known as mind-body healing, for over twenty years. His major training has been with Dr. Lawrence LeShan and Dr. Carl Simonton. He was the principal clinical psychologist at Dr. Contreras' hospital in Tijuana, where he saw over 1,000 cancer patients in a period of six years. His television shows for cancer patients are still being shown on KPBS.

Illness Addressed

Cancer, arthritis, asthma, multiple sclerosis, lupus, and other autoimmune and psychosomatic disorders.

Type of Service Provided

Intensive psychotherapy is the primary modality, since all disorders can be presumed to be psychosomatic until proven otherwise (Andrew Weil, M.D.). Once basic underlying issues are identified and processed using EMDR, Gestalt models, and other specific techniques, then plans are made to create a new life for the patient, a life with meaning, one that "makes us glad to get out of bed in the morning and glad to go to bed at night—the kind of life that makes us look zestfully to each day and to the future."' This kind of life tends to halt and even remit a cancer process. This is the Turning Point (Lawrence LeShan, Ph.D.).

Related Readings

The Psychobiology of Mind-Body Healing by Dr. Ernest Rossi.
Cancer as a Turning Point by Dr. Lawrence LeShan.
Getting Well Again by Dr. Carl Simonton.

Costs

$125 for each ninety-minute session. It is suggested that patients stay at the Optimum Health Institute, which is nearby. (See listing in this book.)

Method of Payment

Cash and checks are accepted.

Resources for Wholeness and Achievement

2522 Boulder Road
Altadena, California 91001
United States

(818) 797-3834
Fax: (818) 798-5815

Contact Person

Arlene Harder.

Primary Personnel

Arlene Harder, M.A., M.F.C.C., certified by the Academy for Guided Imagery.

Directions

Located in Altadena, California, north of Pasadena.

Background

Arlene Harder has seventeen years of experience in the field of imagery and psychotherapy, and is cofounder of The Wellness Community—Foothills, a psychosocial support program for cancer patients and their families. Early in her work as a licensed marriage and family therapist, she realized that the relaxation and imagery techniques she taught her clients not only improved their emotional, mental, and spiritual outlook on life, but also enhanced physical well-being. Although some patients who use Resources for Wholeness and Achievement techniques choose not to follow conventional medicine, many use these techniques to alleviate side effects while undergoing medical treatment.

Illness Addressed

All chronic and life-challenging illnesses, especially cancer.

Type of Program Offered

A two-hour class called "Imagery and the Fight for Recovery" is offered free of charge at The Wellness Community—Foothills, beginning in March and October each year. Patients are given imagery exercises for pain control, stress reduction, enhancing the body's natural healing mechanism, listening to the wisdom of intuition, and uncovering the patient's symbols of hope, love, and health. The fifteen exercises used in the class, plus more than fifteen others, may be ordered by contacting Resources for Wholeness and Achievement. An audio program is being developed to be used in conjunction with exercises taught in the class. Individualized sessions are offered at the office in Altadena to teach patients how to use imagery and stress reduction techniques to fit their particular needs and circumstances, and to explore the emotional and spiritual issues that are part of chronic and life-challenging illness.

Length of Program/Stay

Except for the two-hour, six-week imagery classes, there is no minimum or maximum time a person might want to set aside for using relaxation and imagery techniques in his or her own home. Some patients may wish to come for a few sessions once a week for several weeks. Others may wish to schedule several individualized sessions over a short period of time if they are from out of town or wish to maximize their use of these techniques.

Costs

Cancer patients can receive, at no charge, the tape "Imagery for Cancer Patients: A Gift from Arlene Harder." The first side of the tape provides information on using imagery in the fight for recovery, and the second side has a guided imagery exercise called, Experiencing Medical Procedures as Healing Adventures. In addition, a series of guided imagery exercise tapes is available. Each set contains two tapes with four different imagery exercises. One set is $12.95; two are $19.95. More than two are $8.95 per set. Shipping and handling are additional. To fit each person's unique situation, the sets can be chosen from among five categories: countering life-challenging and chronic illness; achieving and maintaining physical well-being; accomplishing your goals; creating loving relationships; and improving self-confidence. Write, call, or fax for a free list of currently available tapes. Individualized sessions are based on a sliding scale, from $40 to $75 per hour. Out-of-town patients may contact the office for motel recommendations.

Method of Payment

Tapes are sent prepaid by check, money order, or credit card. Payment for sessions is expected at each session. Some insurance is accepted.

Self-Help Groups, Local

Throughout the United States, various self-help groups are available to provide support for individuals and families who are experiencing illnesses and other crises. To locate a self-help group in your area, see National Self-Help Clearinghouse in the Information Services section of this book.

Simonton Cancer Center

P.O. Box 890
Pacific Palisades, California 90272
United States

(800) 459-3424
(310) 457-3811
Fax: (310) 457-0421

Contact Person

Karen Smith, Susan Osti, Inge Finnegan.

Primary Personnel

O. Carl Simonton, M.D.

Directions

Sessions are held at a retreat in Santa Barbara.

Illness Addressed

Cancer.

Type of Service Provided

The center holds five-and-a-half-day retreats for cancer patients. Its program is based on the sucessful model for emotional intervention and support that Dr. Simonton pioneered in the treatment of cancer patients. The program focuses on the influence of beliefs and belief systems. Participants learn techniques for enriching their lives in order to promote their health, lifestyle counseling, and relaxation and mental imagery (creative thinking) exercises. Participants explore the importance of gentleness, the role of stress, secondary gain, and other contributing factors to disease.

Related Readings

Getting Well Again by O. Carl Simonton, M.D., Stephanie Matthews-Simonton, and James Creighton.

The Healing Journey by O. Carl Simonton, M.D.

These and other books and cassette tapes are available through mail order. Call the center's Tapes and Literature Department at 800-338-2360.

Length of Program/Stay

Five-and-a-half days.

Costs

$3,500 for two people.

Method of Payment

Cash, checks, Visa, and MasterCard are accepted. The center does not take insurance assignments.

Smith Farm

1501 32nd Street, N.W.
Washington, D.C. 20007
United States

(202) 338-2330
Fax: (202) 338-2333

Contact Person

Shanti Norris, program director.

Primary Personnel

Michael Lerner, Ph.D., president; Barbara S. Coleman, C.E.O.

Background

Smith Farm brings the Commonweal Cancer Help Program to the Washington area (the program was developed over the last decade at Commonweal by Michael Lerner and Rachel Naomi Remen). Smith Farm was founded in 1986 by Barbara Smith Coleman, an artist dedicated to bringing new resources for the healing arts to this area.

Illness Addressed

All forms of cancer, with additional clinical categories planned for future programs.

Type of Service Provided

Week-long residential, educational (nontreatment) programs for eight participants (and sometimes spouse or support person) who are facing cancer in their lives. This adjunctive support program includes stress reduction, health education, vegetarian diet, and group support to explore issues, choices, and concerns of people with cancer, under the guidance of an experienced and caring staff.

Related Readings

Choices in Healing: Integrating the Best of Conventional and Complementary Approaches to Cancer by Michael Lerner, Ph.D.

Length of Program/Stay

Seven-day residential program.

Costs

$1,480 all-inclusive; some scholarship help may be available.

Method of Payment

Cash or checks are accepted.

Leila Stephens

Santa Barbara, California
United States

(805) 684-7692
(800) 665-8703

Contact Person

Leila Stephens.

Background

Leila Stephens works mostly with the subconscious mind and the physical body, coaching the patient to be the most empowered he or she can be. She teaches patients how to do visualizations, eat healthy foods, eliminate negative beliefs and instill health-affirming beliefs, and clear up emotional problems that stand in the way of health. She also teaches pain control techniques and how to deal with testing and exam phobias. She lectures internationally on the mind-body connection, and teaches these techniques to other therapists and oncologists.

Illness Addressed

Cancer, AIDS, and others.

Type of Service Provided

Individual and group sessions, hypnotherapy, and neurolinguistic programming.

Length of Program/Stay

No specific length of time. The aim of this program is to make the patient independent. After patients learn the techniques, they can do daily visualizations on their own. Follow-up sessions by phone are also possible.

Costs

Free group sessions are held in Santa Barbara once a month. Individual sessions are $150 for fifty minutes.

Method of Payment

No credit cards are accepted. The patient is billed, and may be reimbursed by some insurance companies.

Synergy Seminars

11770 Warner Avenue, Suite 206
Fountain Valley, California 92708
United States

(714) 549-4484

Contact Person

Charles D. Leviton, Ed.D.; Patti Leviton, C.H.T.

Directions

405 freeway to Harbor Boulevard (Costa Mesa). North two miles to Warner. West one-third of a mile.

Background

Synergy Seminars was formed by the Levitons. They conduct lectures, seminars, and week-end retreats, specializing in hypnosis and guided imagery. They believe in the mind-body connection, and that all illnesses have underlying emotional and psychological causes. When these causes are uncovered and addressed appropriately, the body can heal itself or assist in the process. Charles D. Leviton, Ed.D., is a hypnotherapist and a professor at Orange Coast College; he also has twenty-nine years' experience as a marriage and family therapist. Patti Leviton is a certified hypnotherapist and a cancer survivor.

Illness Addressed
Cancer and all other illnesses.

Type of Service Provided
Psychotherapy and hypnotherapy—no medical service of any kind.

Related Readings
There Is No Bad Truth: The Search for Self by C.D. Leviton. Ed.D. Kendall-Hunt Publications, 1990.

Length of Program/Stay
Outpatient and weekend retreats from 9:00 a.m. Friday to noon Sunday.

Costs
$250 for weekend: two nights' lodging, three meals, and fifteen-hour workshop—seminar included.

Method of Payment
Cash or checks are accepted. Insurance accepted for psychotherapy.

Colin Tipping, M.Ed., DipH.

26 Briar Gate Lane
Marietta, Georgia 30066
United States

(770) 428-9228
Internet: www.althealing.org
E-mail: colint@mindspring.com

Contact Person
Colin Tipping, M.Ed. DipH.

Primary Personnel

Colin Tipping, M.Ed. DipH., Certified Hypnotherapist.

Background

Colin Tipping, is cofounder and director of The Georgia CancerHelp Program. He is an experienced teacher, counselor, hypnotherapist, minister, author, and workshop facilitator. Colin has an honors degree in Education from London University, where he taught for ten years before emigrating to the United States in 1984. He worked for five years as a corporate EAP counselor. He studied with Lawrence LeShan, Jeanne Achterberg, and Frank Lawliss for professional certification in working with people with life-threatening illness.

Illness Addressed

Primarily cancer, as well as any illness for which healing imagery is appropriate.

Type of Program Offered

Golden Key Healing Tapes—custom healing imagery tapes. Patients can schedule a thirty-minute telephone conversation with Colin. He will then craft a special tape for that person, and follow up with others as progress is made.

Related Readings

Books by Jeanne Achterberg and Belleruth Naperstek et.al.

Length of Program/Stay

Variable as required.

Costs

$175 for a thirty-minute consultation and the custom tape.

Method of Payment

Cash or checks are accepted.

Virginia Veach, Ph.D., M.F.C.C., P.T.

Ting-Sha Institute
P.O. Box 266
Point Reyes Station, California 94956
United States

(415) 663-1190

Primary Personnel

Virginia Veach, Ph.D., M.F.C.C., P.T., also an ordained minister and director of the Ting-Sha Institute.

Background

In addition to an office in Point Reyes Station, Dr. Veach has an office in San Rafael. She became a physical therapist in 1955 and a psychotherapist in 1972. She is also a licensed marriage, family, and child therapist, and an ordained minister. She has been a co-leader with the Commonweal Cancer Help Program retreats since their inception. Ting-Sha Institute is a nonprofit educational corporation founded in order to demonstrate that medicine, art, psychotherapy, and spiritual practices need not be isolated from each other; to establish a center that offers educational programs for professionals and the general public; and to encourage a holistic approach to social action. Ting-Sha has offered classes, seminars, and retreats since 1972.

Illness Addressed

Cancer, heart disease, autoimmune diseases (such as lupus, rheumatoid arthritis, and environmental diseases), and other chronic and acute illnesses.

Type of Service Provided

Chronic and critical illness counseling, transpersonal psychotherapy, family therapy, art therapy, touch, pain control, stress reduction, physical therapy education, visualization, and week-long retreats for cancer patients and health professionals. These retreats include gentle stretching and movement, sensory awareness, meditation, creativity, vegetarian meals, access to information about complementary therapies, and time to explore the beautiful surroundings.

Related Readings

You Can Fight for Your Life by Lawrence LeShan. M. Evans and Co., 1977.
Cancer, Another Way? by Ainslie Meares, M.D.
Cancer and Vitamin C by Ewan Cameron and Linus Pauling. Linus Pauling Institute of Science and Medicine, 1979.

Length of Program/Stay

Week-long retreats.

Costs

The all-inclusive basic fee for the retreat is $1,550 per person. A $250 deposit is required before arrival. Each seminar is limited to nine participants; spouses and other close support people are welcome to enroll at the same fee and with the same full program as the other participants. Individual counseling: $100 for one hour; family counseling: $125 for one hour.

Method of Payment

Cash or checks are accepted.

Well Being International Inc.

P.O. Box 1277
Haiku, Maui, Hawaii 96708
United States

(808) 572-2300
(808) 573-1414
Fax: (808) 573-1414

Contact Person

Fredrick R. Honig or Meenakshi P. Honig, codirectors.

Primary Personnel

Fredrick R. Honig and Meenakshi P. Honig, certified instructors of integral yoga and stress management consultants.

Directions

Twenty-five minutes from Kahului Airport, Maui. Please call for directions.

Background

Well Being International Inc. is a nonprofit organization dedicated to individual and global peace, health, and harmony. The facility, which offers programs and products for well-being, includes a guest house on an eleven-acre oceanfront nature sanctuary with a waterfall.

Illness Addressed

The facility's health-enhancing programs and products, based on balanced lifestyle choices, can benefit patients with cancer, heart disease, and other disorders.

Type of Service Provided

Stress management, yoga, meditation, goals clarification, nutritional guidance, healthy back care, nature exercise therapy, massage therapy, and balanced lifestyle management.

Related Readings

The books of Dr. Dean Ornish, whose program is based on integral yoga, which we teach.

Length of Program/Stay

The length of stay is tailored to the needs and wishes of the individual.

Costs

Because we customize our programs to meet the needs of the individual, costs vary. Programs are tailored to work in harmony with the financial considerations of the individual, ranging from economy to deluxe.

Method of Payment

Cash, checks, traveler's checks, Visa, and MasterCard are accepted. Insurance is not accepted.

The Wellness Community

2716 Ocean Park Boulevard
Santa Monica, California 90405
United States

(310) 314-2555
Fax: (310) 314-7586

Primary Personnel

TWC-National: Harold H. Benjamin, Ph.D., founder and president; Mitch Golant, Ph.D., vice president program; Michael States, M.F.C.C., program director, TWC-National Training Center.

Directions

Call individual locations for directions.

Background

Established in 1982, The Wellness Community (TWC) is a free, multidimensional, non-residential program of psychological and emotional support for cancer patients and families as an adjunct to conventional treatment. The heart of the program is the "Patient Active Concept," which states that if cancer patients participate in their fight for recovery along with their physicians, they will improve the quality of their lives and enhance the possibility of recovery. Program services, philosophy, and methodology are consistent throughout all TWC facilities. Each TWC is financially autonomous from the national organization. All funds remain within the local community. Since 1982, The Wellness Community has helped over 30,000 cancer patients.

Illness Addressed

The Wellness Community has as its sole focus, cancer patients and families fighting for recovery.

Type of Service Provided

Ongoing support groups, site-specific networking groups, workshops, lectures and physician lectures, stress reduction, relaxation/visualization series to trigger the relaxation response, and social events and parties where people with cancer and their families learn they can go on living their lives despite a diagnosis of cancer. All groups are facilitated by specially trained, licensed psychotherapists.

Related Readings

The Wellness Community Guide to Fighting for Recovery by Harold Benjamin, Ph.D. Putnam, 1995.

From Victim to Victor by Harold Benjamin, Ph.D. Jeremy P. Tarcher, Inc.-Dell, 1987.

Minding the Body, Mending the Mind by Joan Boryshenko, Ph.D.

Helping Yourself Help Others by Rosalyn Carter, Susan Golant.

Relaxation Response by Herbert Benson, M.D.

Living Beyond Your Limits by David Spiegel, M.D.

Length of Program/Stay

Ongoing, for as long as someone is engaged in the fight for recovery.

Costs

All programs are without charge to participants.

Its national headquarters is in Santa Monica, California, but The Wellness Community can also be contacted at its several other locations (all in the United States):

Baltimore:
Dulaney Center II
901 Dulaney Valley Road, #710
Baltimore, Maryland 21204
(410) 832-2719
Fax: (410) 337-0937

Greater Boston:
1320 Centre Street, #305
Newton Centre, Massachusetts 02159
(617) 332-1919
Fax: (617) 332-2727

Greater Cincinnati:
Bank One Towers
8044 Montgomery Road, #385
Cincinnati, Ohio 45236
(513) 791-4060
Fax: (513) 791-8239

Delaware:
1526 Gilpin Avenue
Wilmington, Delaware 19806
(302) 656-8410
Fax: (302) 656-5547

Southwest Florida:
3900 Clark Road, Building P3
Sarasota, Florida 34233
(941) 921-5539
Fax: (941) 921-5061

Foothills:
200 E. Del Mar, Suite 118
Pasadena, California 91105
(818) 796-1083
Fax: (818) 796-0601

Central Indiana:
9465 Keystone Crossing, #145
Indianapolis, Indiana 46240
(317) 257-1505
Fax: (317) 254-4534

Knoxville:
1844 Terrace Avenue
Knoxville, Tennessee 37916
(423) 546-4661
Fax: (423) 522-1912

Northwest Ohio:
5565 Airport Highway, Suite 100
Toledo, Ohio 43615
(419) 861-HOPE (4673)
(419) 872-2070
Fax: (419) 861-0776

Philadelphia:
4610 City Line Avenue
Philadelphia, Pennsylvania 19131
(215) 879-7733
Fax: (215) 879-6575

Greater St. Louis:
10425 Old Olive Street Road, Suite 202
St. Louis, Missouri 63141
(314) 993-4333
Fax: (314) 993-6835

San Diego:
8555 Aero Drive, #340
San Diego, California 92123
(619) 467-1065
Fax: (619) 467-1082

S.F. East Bay:
1777 N. California, Suite #200
Walnut Creek, California 94596
(510) 933-0107
Fax: (510) 933-0249

South Bay Cities:
109 W. Torrance Boulevard, #100
Redondo Beach, California 90277
(310) 376-3550
Fax: (310) 372-2904

Valley/Ventura:
530 Hampshire Road
Westlake Village, California 91361
(805) 379-4777
Fax: (805) 371-6231

Wellness House

131 North County Line Road
Hinsdale, Illinois 60521-2401
United States

(630) 323-5150
Fax: (630) 654-5346

Contact Person

William E. Walker, Ph.D., executive director; Paul R. Ginter, Ed.D., program director.

Primary Personnel

William E. Walker, Ph.D.; Paul R. Ginter, Ed.D.; Tim Tumlin, Ph.D., assessment director; Jeanne Cella, M.S., associate program director.

Directions

From 294 (either northbound or southbound), exit Ogden West, cross two lanes of traffic and make a left on County Line Road. Proceed south for six blocks. Wellness House is on the southeast corner of County Line and Walnut. Can also use Chicago-Aurora Metro Line—Highlands stop.

Background

Wellness House is a not-for-profit organization that provides encouragement, education, and emotional support for people wanting to maintain or enhance their quality of life through the cancer experience. Wellness House is not affiliated with any hospital, but works with other health care organizations to provide comprehensive services. The programming helps cancer patients discover specific needs and develop the personal resources to meet them. Wellness House currently sees 400 people each week.

Illness Addressed

Cancer, and the challenges presented for those whose lives are complicated by the cancer of a loved one.

Type of Service Provided

Weekly committed groups include those providing primarily emotional support, and those with a greater psychoeducational emphasis. The Positively Wellness series provides daily classes, including tai chi, yoga, assertiveness, meditation, qi gong, and fitness. Special-interest groups focus specifically on issues related to ovarian, multiple myeloma, and breast cancer, and children whose parents have cancer. Additionally, weekly lectures cover a wide range of concerns regarding the cancer experience.

Related Readings

Healing and the Mind by Bill Moyers. New York: Doubleday, 1993.

Full Catastrophe Living: Using the Wisdom of Your Body and Mind to Face Stress, Pain, and Illness by J. Kabat-Zinn. New York: Doubleday, 1990.

Effect of Psychosocial Treatment on Survival of Patients With Metastatic Breast Cancer by Spiegl, et al. *The Lancet* 888-891, 1989.

A Structured Psychiatric Intervention for Cancer Patients, Changes Over Time in Immunological Measures by Fawzy, et al. *Archives of General Psychiatry* 47-729-735, 1990.

Triumph: Getting Back to Normal When You Have Cancer by Marion Morra and Eve Potts. Avon Books, 1990.

Support Plus, A Manual for Wellness House by William E. Walker, et al., Wellness House, 1996.

Length of Program/Stay

Groups/programs are offered on a quarterly basis, including both committed and drop-in sessions.

Costs

None.

Wellspring Foundation of New England, Inc.

P.O. Box 317
Lyme, New Hampshire 03768
United States

(603) 795-2144
Fax: (603) 795-2155

Contact Person

Deb Steele, program director; Don Dickey, executive director.

Primary Personnel

Donald Dickey, J.D., executive director; Deborah Steele, M.Ed., program director.

Directions

The Wellspring Foundation holds its five-day cancer retreats at the Gove Hill Conference Center in Thetford, Vermont, Exit 14 off I-91. Complete directions are provided with acceptance of application.

Background

The Wellspring Foundation was started by Dr. Robert M. Rufsvold, a family physician, in 1994. Its mission includes a committment to helping people with chronic illness seek physical, psychological, emotional, and spiritual healing. The foundation is indebted to the Commonweal Cancer Help Program of Bolinas, California, as its role model and guide in setting up and running its retreats.

Illness Addressed

Wellspring addresses the experience of having cancer on a physical, emotional, mental, and spiritual level. It discusses conventional and alternative—i.e., complementary— therapies, and offers the services below. Adults with any stage of cancer who are under the care of a physician, are welcome.

Type of Service Provided

Five-day retreat offering daily yoga, meditation, and group sessions that address the experience of having cancer. Vegetarian food is provided—also individual sand tray and art therapy, nutritional counseling with a naturopathic doctor, massages, Reiki, meeting with a medical doctor, and a full evening program with music, writing, and discussion.

Related Readings

Choices in Healing by Michael Lerner.

Length of Program/Stay

Retreat lasts five days—Sunday afternoon until Friday afternoon. Retreats are held approximately every eight weeks (six to eight times a year).

Costs

$1,500 per participant for five days. Some scholarship money is available.

Method of Payment

Cash or checks are accepted. Insurance coverage is limited—ask your insurer ahead of time. The foundation is working on getting acceptance from HMOs.

SUPPORT PROGRAMS

Overseas (Australia, United Kingdom)

Cancer Support Association Inc.

80 Railway Street
Cottesloe (Perth)
Western Australia 6011
Australia

011-61-09-384-3544
Fax: 011-61-09-384-6196

Contact Person

Pam Ryan.

Primary Personnel

Bill Smith, president; Ellen Levett, secretary; Angela Tillier, center director.

Directions

The association is located in Cottesloe, a suburb of Perth, the capital city of the state of Western Australia.

Background

The Cancer Support Association was formed and incorporated in 1984. Its objectives are to assist cancer patients and their families; to engage in public education programs for cancer patients and their families; to improve the quality and length of life for the cancer patient in a manner both complementary and supplementary to prescribed medical treatments; to provide active support for cancer patients and their families to help them recognize the importance of their personal contribution in fighting and overcoming cancer; and to encourage those with cancer to accept responsibility for the quality of their lives by paying particular attention to the holistic approach of self-care, which includes meditation, positive thinking, diet and nutrition, and related subjects.

Illness Addressed

Cancer.

Type of Service Provided

Wellness course, support groups, counseling, art therapy, meditation, tai chi, massage, and access to a large resource library containing information on all types of cancer treatments.

Costs

The association is a nonprofit organization. All income is derived from donations, fundraising activities, and bequests, and is strictly applied toward fulfilling the association's aims and objectives.

Method of Payment

Cash, checks, and credit cards are accepted.

Hereford Cancer Help Clinic

Brookfield
Tarrington
Herefordshire HR1.4HZ
England
United Kingdom

011-44-432-890341
Fax: 011-44-432-890792

20 Castle Street
Tredegar
Gwent NP2 3DF
Wales
United Kingdom

Primary Personnel

Richard Lamerton, M.D., Hospice of the Marches.

Directions

Exit 2 from M50. A417 to Ledbury. A438 (Hereford Road) to Tarrington.

Background

Hereford Cancer Help Clinic is under the auspices of the Hospice of the Marches. For terminally ill patients, there is no discontinuity of care. This is not an inpatient facility. The staff visits people's homes as often as necessary. The clinic is open every Friday.

Illness Addressed

Cancer, AIDS, leukemia, amyotrophic lateral sclerosis, Parkinson's disease, and others.

Type of Service Provided

The clinic gives advice on diet and nutrition; provides a personal interview with a counselor; and uses healing and relaxation techniques such as acupuncture, massage, osteopathy, yoga, art therapy, counseling, hypnotherapy, and conventional therapy.

Related Readings

The clinic will provide upon request information regarding past patients.

Costs

A day's care in one of the clinics costs about £50 per patient. This includes therapist's fees, the Bristol Diet lunch, and rent of the building. However, no payment is required. Funds are raised by appeals, street collections, garage sales, etc. Patients may make a voluntary donation.

Plymouth Natural Health and Healing Centre

100 Lipson Road
Lipson
Plymouth
Devon PL4 8RJ
England
United Kingdom

Plymouth 228785
Plymouth 660712
Cornwood 383

Contact Person

Gillian Fordham, chairman.

Primary Personnel

Dr. Alec Forbes, president; Dr. Adrian White, vice president; Frank Smale, vice president.

Background

Founded in 1977, the centre is a registered charity affiliated with Bristol Cancer Help Centre, National Federation of Spiritual Healers, LIFE Cancer Centre, and LIFE Foundation. Its aim is to help people help themselves. It is staffed entirely by volunteers. The centre is open Monday to Friday from 11:00 a.m. to 4:00 p.m.

Illness Addressed

Cancer and any other form of ill health.

Type of Service Provided

Counseling, healing, relaxation, visualization, meditation, reflexology, yoga, osteopathy, homeopathy, shiatsu massage, and nutritional advice. Patients learn how to release and mobilize inner resources of self-healing.

Costs

Donation.

Relaxation Centre of Queensland, Limited

Corner of Brookes and Wickham Streets
Fortitude Valley
Brisbane 4006
Queensland
Australia

011-07-3854-1986
Fax: 011-07-3252-7408

Contact Person

Marge Garrett or Lionel Fifield.

Primary Personnel

Lionel Fifield; Marge Garrett; Bert Weir.

Directions

Corner of Brookes and Wickham Streets, one mile from the center of Brisbane.

Background

The centre was established in 1974, a result of the desire of several people to make a centre available with numerous supportive courses, workshops and materials, to which all people would have access, whatever their financial means.

Illness Addressed

No specific illness is addressed. The interest is in helping people be more responsible for their lives, and be aware of their inner resources.

Type of Service Provided

Courses, seminars, one-to-one relaxation, books, tapes, library, and individual appointments.

Length of Program/Stay

Involvement according to the needs of the individual. The program is nonresidential.

Costs

Fees are acknowledged as very low, and are always negotiable.

Method of Payment

Cash or checks are accepted.

Thorpe Bay Self-Help Cancer Group

22 St. James Avenue
Thorpe Bay
Southend-on-Sea
Essex SS1 3LH
England
United Kingdom

011-0702-584111
011-0702-587640

Contact Person

Angela Ekers or Maureen Holmes.

Primary Personnel

Angela Ekers.

Background

The group's aim is to give support to people who have cancer and to their families. Angela Ekers is a member of the National Federation of Spiritual Healers Association. The group is registered with Bacup and CancerLink.

Illness Addressed
Cancer.

Type of Service Provided

The group meets in an informal atmosphere every Friday at 7:00 p.m. The group provides a way for sharing problems and information; the teaching of relaxation, meditation, and positive thinking; the use of a library with books and tapes; art therapy; dietary help; refreshments; a way to make new friends; and, if desired, spiritual healing.

Costs

Costs not submitted for publication.

INFORMATION SERVICES

North America (United States)

Arlin J. Brown Information Center Inc.

P.O. Box 251
Fort Belvoir, Virginia 22060
United States

(540) 752-9511

Directions

Contact by mail and phone only.

Background

Founded in February 1963 as an information organization, the Arlin Brown Center investigates nontoxic cancer therapies. It publishes a newsletter that includes questions and answers by leading specialists. This group has proposed a national health freedom bill to allow Americans to use any type of remedy they choose. The center was the first cancer organization in the United States devoted to nontoxic treatments. This is an information center only.

Illness Addressed

Cancer.

Type of Information Offered

Information on different types of cancer, health methods, degenerative diseases, and nontoxic cancer therapies.

Related Readings

March of Truth on Cancer.
Health Victory Bulletin.
Monthly newsletter.
The center also offers a mail-order book list upon request.

Costs

Member for one year: $25. Contributing member for one year: $35. Supporting member for two years: $80. Supporting member for five years: $200. Life member: $500. Perpetual member: $1,000.

Method of Payment

Cash and checks are accepted.

Cancer Control Society and Cancer Book House

2043 North Berendo Street
Los Angeles, California 90027
United States

(213) 663-7801

Contact Person

Lorraine Rosenthal.

Directions

Interstate 5 to Los Feliz off ramp. Go west for about one mile to North Berendo, turn left, and go one-and-a-half blocks. Or else take Hollywood Freeway (101) to Vermont off ramp, go north about one-and-a-half miles to Franklin, turn left, then go two blocks to North Berendo and turn right.

Background

This is an informational and educational nonprofit organization. The Cancer Control Society Convention, held in Los Angeles during the Labor Day weekend, has been the largest gathering of its kind for over twenty years. The purpose of the society is public education in the prevention and control of cancer and other diseases through nutrition, tests, and nontoxic alternative therapies (such as laetrile, Gerson, Hoxsey, Koch, enzymes, immunotherapy, wheatgrass, herbs, megavitamins and minerals, and detoxification). The society was originally the Los Angeles chapter of Cancer Victims and Friends from 1966 to 1972. In 1973, it became the Cancer Control Society.

Illness Addressed

Cancer, diabetes, arthritis, multiple sclerosis, and heart disease.

Type of Information Offered

An information set, a clinic directory, a list of patients, books, videos, and a list of clinic tours. The society also offers a bookstore that has a comprehensive mail-order list; conventions; and the *Cancer Control Journal*, which it publishes.

Related Readings

An extensive list is available of books and reprints on cancer and other nutrition-related diseases. Films and videos are also available.

Costs

Yearly membership: $25. Information set $10. Information set plus a sample issue of *Cancer Control Journal: $15.*

Method of Payment

Money orders, checks, and credit cards are accepted. Insurance is not accepted.

Cancer Prevention Coalition

520 North Michigan Avenue, Suite 410
Chicago, Illinois 60611
United States

(312) 467-0600
Fax: (312) 467-0599

Contact Person

Melissa Troester, M.S., program director.

Primary Personnel

Dr. Samuel S. Epstein, M.D., chairman.

Directions

Located in downtown Chicago on the corner of Michigan Avenue and Grand Avenue.

Background

The Cancer Prevention Coalition, which opened Chicago offices in 1994, grew out of a February 1992 press conference in Washington, D.C., where more than sixty leading experts in cancer prevention and public health warned that the United States was losing the war against cancer. An overemphasis on the diagnosis and treatment of cancer and relative neglect of its prevention, coupled with ineffective regulation of carcinogens in air, water, food, and consumer products, has substantially contributed to escalating cancer rates and an annual death toll over 500,000. The Cancer Prevention Coalition is implementing community-based solutions for the reduction of avoidable cancer risks. Local grassroots activities are designed to increase awareness and stimulate action for cancer prevention. CPC's national advocacy and public policy initiatives are designed to prioritize the role of prevention in federal cancer policies, which in turn will strongly impact at the community level.

Illness Addressed

Cancer prevention, toxic-use reduction, and environmental illnesses.

Type of Information Offered

Cancer Prevention Alerts, Cancer Prevention News, and scientific articles related to avoidable exposures to cancer-causing chemicals.

Related Readings

Cancer Wars by Robert Proctor. Basic Books, 1995.

Politics of Cancer by Samuel S. Epstein, M.D. Sierra Club Books, 1978.

Safe Shopper's Bible by Epstein and Steinman. McMillan Publishing, 1995.

Cancer Prevention News, a quarterly mini-magazine that contains information on how to reduce exposure to cancer-causing chemicals and news on the federal and international regulation of cancer-causing substances.

Costs

Publication lists and costs are available on request. All donations are appreciated and are tax-deductible. Individual memberships start at $35; health professional memberships start at $100.

Method of Payment

Checks and money orders are accepted.

CanHelp

3111 Paradise Bay Road
Port Ludlow, Washington 98365-9771
United States

(206) 437-2291

Primary Personnel

Patrick M. McGrady Jr., founder and director; Dorris Stellner, assistant director.

Background

Mr. McGrady is a medical writer with a talent for translating medical jargon into plain English. A former *Newsweek* Moscow bureau chief, he wrote *The Youth Doctors* and *The Love Doctors* and co-authored *The Pritikin Program for Diet & Exercise* and *Life Zones.* He founded CanHelp to provide clients with up-to-date information on both conventional and alternative therapies. He is not a doctor and does not prescribe therapies. Call first, or send a stamped, self-addressed envelope for free literature.

Illness Addressed
Cancer in all its forms.

Type of Information Offered
After analyzing the patient's medical records and questions and consulting with its own specialists, CanHelp writes an evaluative and detailed report on those alternative, orthodox, and experimental therapies that would appear to offer its client the most promise. The report (five to fifteen pages) covers such matters as content of treatment, length of stay, location, quality of care, costs, phone numbers, personality of physician, and caveats, if any. Accompanying the report are background articles about recommended physicians and treatments and up-to-date computer printouts of relevant studies from CancerLit and other computer medical databases. CanHelp also answers brief follow-up questions and assists in solving logistical problems. The service is available seven days a week, twenty-four hours a day. Reports are sent by express mail, usually within seven working days of receipt of medical records. In emergencies, reports can be completed in as few as two days and sent to the client via fax or modem.

Costs
$400 for seven-day personal report. $100 U.S. extra for foreign-based client's report. $150 extra for emergency two-day personal report.

Method of Payment
A check payable to "CanHelp" should be sent with the medical records.

Center for Advancement in Cancer Education

300 East Lancaster Avenue, Suite 100
Wynnewood, Pennsylvania 19096
United States

(610) 642-4810

Contact Person

Susan Silberstein, Ph.D., executive director.

Directions

Two miles west of intersection of Routes 1 and 30, in the western Philadelphia suburbs.

Background

The center is a nonprofit cancer information, counseling, and referral service, focusing on combining the body's natural healing potential with advances in medical science. Specializing in immune support through clinical nutrition, botanical medicine, and psychoneuroimmunology, the center offers resources for nontoxic approaches as adjuncts or alternatives to conventional treatments. The center has provided educational and consulting services to thousands of health professionals and their patients since 1977.

Illness Addressed

Cancer.

Type of Information Offered

Books, magazines, printed matter, and tapes, as well as private, individualized consultations and referrals to health professionals. Reference library. Classes, seminars, and conferences.

Costs

Books, tapes, and other materials are available at list price or for a nominal fee. Individualized consultations are available to center members at no charge (tax-deductible donation).

Method of Payment

Cash, checks, Visa, and MasterCard are accepted.

Center for Science in the Public Interest

1875 Connecticut Avenue N.W.
Suite 300
Washington, D.C. 20009-5728
United States

(202) 332-9110
Fax: (202) 265-4954

Contact Person

Publications department or nutrition department.

Primary Personnel

Michael Jacobson, Ph.D, executive director.

Directions

Take the Washington Metro subway's Red line to the Dupont Circle stop, use the Q Street exit, go three blocks up Connecticut Avenue to the intersection of Connecticut Avenue and T Street, just before the Washington Hilton hotel. The center is in the Universal North building.

Background

Center for Science in the Public Interest (CSPI) is the nation's leading consumer group concerned with food and nutrition issues. CSPI focuses on diseases that result from consuming too many calories; too much fat, sodium, and sugar; and not enough fiber. CSPI has 750,000 members.

Illness Addressed

Cancer and heart disease.

Type of Information Offered

All CSPI members receive the *Nutrition Action Healthletter,* which takes a self-help and consumer advocacy perspective to address the prevention of cancer and heart disease. A list of other publications will be sent on request.

Costs

Membership for one year is $24 for United States residents and $32 for everyone else. Membership includes a subscription to *Nutrition Action Healthletter* (published ten times a year), and a 10 percent discount on the purchase of various publications.

Method of Payment

Personal checks, money orders, Visa, and MasterCard are accepted on United States orders. Visa, MasterCard, and postal orders (in United States funds) are the only methods accepted on foreign orders.

Committee for Freedom of Choice in Medicine Inc.

1180 Walnut Avenue
Chula Vista, California 91911
United States

(619) 429-8200

Primary Personnel

Robert Bradford; Michael Culbert.

Background

This is a lobbying group that publishes a quarterly newsmagazine called *The Choice*, as well as special reports. This group is headed by the people in charge of American Biologics Hospital in Tijuana, Mexico. It is the successor to the Committee for Freedom of Choice in Cancer Therapy Inc., which was formed in 1974.

Illness Addressed

Chronic systemic metabolic dysfunctions.

Type of Information Offered

The Choice, a quarterly newsmagazine; mail-order supplements; and special reports.

Costs

$16 for a one-year subscription.

Method of Payment

Cash, checks, money orders, American Express, Discover, MasterCard, and Visa are accepted.

Cypress Consultants

2780 East Fowler Avenue
Suite 159
Tampa, Florida 33612-6297
United States

(813) 930-9638
Fax: (813) 930-9596

Contact Person

Dennis Stoltzfoos.

Background

Dennis Stoltzfoos' mother had cancer in 1991. Since then, he has been helping her and others go wherever they need to go for help. He has also spent six years in the Emergency Medical Services, and now teaches nutritional seminars around the country. He believes in and teaches prevention, but constantly meets people with cancer, and refers them to various places around the country and in Mexico for help.

Illness Addressed

Cancer.

Type Information Offered

Information about various cancer clinics. Cypress Consultants has performed the research and visited the clinics, and does its best to match the patient's situation with the place that can offer the most help.

Costs

On an individual basis, but usually no charge.

Foundation for Advancement in Cancer Therapy (FACT)

P.O. Box 1242
Old Chelsea Station
New York, New York 10113
United States

(212) 741-2790

Contact Person

Ruth Sackman.

Background

This nonprofit educational organization serves as a clearinghouse for information about cancer prevention and nontoxic therapies for cancer.

Illness Addressed

Cancer.

Type of Information Offered

FACT believes in the "total person approach," which involves early noninvasive diagnosis, nutrition, detoxification, structural balance, and therapies involving the mind-body connection. Some types of therapy are fever, immuno, cellular, and botanical.

Related Readings

Mail-order books, articles, and cassette tapes are available.

Costs

Any contribution is accepted. For $10 a year, you will receive a subscription to *Cancer Forum,* a FACT publication.

Method of Payment

Cash, checks, and money orders are accepted.

Healing Alternatives Network

1227 San Miguel Avenue
Santa Barbara, California 93109
United States

(805) 564-1229

Contact Person

Suzanne Riordan.

Background

Healing Alternatives Network was formed out of the determination of two women to alleviate the anguish and confusion faced by many people when they are diagnosed with a life-threatening illness. The network recognizes the precious opportunity a health crisis offers to reevaluate the meaning of life and death, and to honor love and all that is sacred. Its aim is to offer prompt and efficient assistance to the individual and his or her family in making the wisest choice among a variety of treatment modalities that address the whole person.

Type of Information Offered

Referral to a variety of information services and treatment providers with an emphasis on healers who are skilled in addressing the mind/body/spirit/emotions connection.

Costs

$25 for a yearly membership entitling one to a quarterly newsletter showcasing promising healers and holisitc treatment centers. $50 for up to thirty minutes or $75 for thirty-one- to sixty-minute consultations for referral.

Method of Payment

Checks or money orders are accepted for membership. Money orders are accepted for telephone consultations.

Healing Choices Cancer Report Service

144 Saint John's Place
Brooklyn, New York 11217
United States

(718) 636-4433

Contact Person

Anne Beattie, coordinator.

Primary Personnel

Ralph W. Moss, Ph.D., writer; Anne Beattie, M.A., L.M.Th., coordinator.

Background

Ralph W. Moss, Ph.D., is an internationally acclaimed science writer who has spent more than twenty years investigating and writing about cancer issues. He is the author of *Cancer Therapy, Questioning Chemotherapy,* and *The Cancer Industry.* Since 1991, he has been an advisor to the National Institutes of Health's Office of Alternative Medicine.

Illness Addressed

Cancer.

Type of Information Offered

The Healing Choices report provides the patient with objective, detailed information on the most promising alternative methods and practitioners for the particular type of cancer being faced. Reports are forty to sixty pages long.

Costs

The fee is $275. This includes the report, next-day delivery, and any follow-up questions the patient may have after receiving the report.

Method of Payment

Checks, money orders, Visa, MasterCard, and American Express are accepted.

Health, Research, and Referral Center

1442 Mendelssohn Drive
Westlake, Ohio 44145
United States

(216) 835-2025

Contact Person

Dr. Jan Petrik.

Primary Personnel

Dr. Jan Petrik; John Petrik.

Background

Jan Petrik, president of the center, is a Naturopathic Doctor with a Ph.D. in Nutrition. She has studied nutrition and preventive health care extensively for many years, and works in conjunction with various medical professionals in the holistic field. She and her staff have traveled extensively to numerous parts of the world researching holistic clinics and alternative therapies.

Illness Addressed

Cancer and all diseases.

Type of Information Offered

The center maintains an extensive computer database of expert doctors, researchers, and scientists from around the world, who are the best and most respected in their field of expertise. Daily contact with these doctors and scientists enables the center to provide the most up-to-date research available for doctors, patients, and referrals. Consultations, comprehensive research data for various illnesses, referrals, and tour guide services can be provided at a nominal cost.

Costs

Costs vary, depending on the type and extent of the service.

The Health Resource, Inc.

564 Locust Street
Conway, Arkansas 72032
United States

(501) 329-5272
(800) 949-0090
Fax: (501) 329-9489
Internet: http://www.thehealthresource.com
E-mail: moreinfo@thehealthresource.com

Contact Person

Jan Guthrie.

Primary Personnel

A staff of nine, including four researchers who are highly trained in accessing medical information.

Background

The Health Resource, Inc., was established in 1984 as a result of founder/director Janice Guthrie's bout with cancer. She extensively researched her rare type of ovarian cancer. She relates, "The information I gathered helped me to locate a physician who had special interest in treating my cancer, and enabled me to be an active participant with him in the decisions regarding my treatment. My research was so important in helping me to regain a sense of control over my personal health, that I decided to do similar research as a service for others with medical problems." Guthrie and her staff are committed to helping patients survey all their treatment options—including conventional, experimental, and alternative. Their goal is "not to leave a stone unturned" in finding effective treatment options for their clients. Guthrie participated in the United States Congressional study of alternative cancer therapies in 1990.

Illness Addressed

Any medical condition, including all types of cancer.

Type of Information Offered

Clients receive an individualized, comprehensive report on their specific medical condition. This report contains information on the latest treatment options—conventional, experimental, and alternative—and on current research, nutrition, top conventional specialists and holistic practitioners, and resource organizations. The report includes a bibliography with summaries of articles plus copies of medical journal articles and excerpts from publications. The researcher highlights the report to guide readers to information that addresses their questions and is relevant to their condition. Reports also contain: profiles of patients with the same type of cancer who either recovered or outlived their life expectancy; copies of the computer search of the international cancer literature for information on the latest treatments and research for the client's cancer; a list of clinical trials (experimental therapies) for their type of cancer; information on the alternative practitioners and clinics that The Health Resource considers to be reputable, and that have had success in treating the client's cancer; a list of outstanding specialists in the treatment of their type of cancer; tips for coping effectively with chemotherapy and radiation therapy, including information on nutritional and herbal supplements that may be helpful during treatments; and ways to stimulate the immune system.

Costs

Individualized reports on cancer are $350 plus shipping. Reports on noncancer conditions are $250 plus shipping. Reports are shipped within three to five working days; emergency one- to two-day service is $75 extra. Clients receive, at no charge, news bulletins about significant new treatments for their condition, and The Health Resource biannual newsletter. Clients are also offered an update service (for a fee). Reports carry a full money-back guarantee.

Method of Payment

Checks, money orders, Visa, MasterCard, Discover, and American Express are accepted. To order, please call and speak directly with one of our researchers, so that he or she can obtain a full medical history from you.

International Academy of Nutrition and Preventive Medicine

34 Wall Street, Suite 405
Asheville, North Carolina 28801
United States

(704) 258-3243
Fax: (704) 254-2286

P.O. Box 18433
Asheville, North Carolina 28814
United States

Contact Person

Elizabeth A. Pavka, M.S., L.N., director.

Primary Personnel

Whitney J. Ponder, office manager.

Background

The International Academy of Nutrition and Preventive Medicine was incorporated in 1987 from a merger of the International College of Applied Nutrition, founded in 1936, with the International Academy of Preventive Medicine, founded in 1970. The purpose of IANPM is to advance the broadest goals of health and preventive medicine among health professionals and the public. These goals include encouraging research on the relation of nutrition to health and the prevention of disease; dissemination of knowledge about health and prevention; and encouraging a focus on nutrition, health, and preventive medicine in medical education and among practicing physicians, dentists, optometrists, chiropractors, nutritionists, and other health professionals. IANPM also encourages and invites coordination with other professional and lay organizations with similar purposes.

Illness Addressed

All degenerative diseases.

Type of Information Offered

Information about professional members who use nutrition for all degenerative conditions; newsletter; *Journal of Applied Nutrition*.

Related Readings

Your Health, newsletter.
Journal of Applied Nutrition.

Costs

Friends membership: $30 per year. Professional membership: $150 per year. Journal subscription: $85 (United States), $110 (foreign).

Method of Payment

Cash, checks, or money orders are accepted.

International Association of Cancer Victors and Friends

7740 West Manchester Avenue #110
Playa del Rey, California 90293
United States

(213) 822-5032

Primary Personnel

Frank Cousineau, president; Ann Cinquina, editor of *Cancer Victors Journal*.

Background

Founded in 1963 by Cecile Hoffman in San Diego, this association was created as an information organization specifically emphasizing nontoxic cancer therapies. An educational nonprofit corporation, the IACVF disseminates information concerning alternative cancer therapies. It reports on the most recent cancer studies and treatments. *Cancer Victors Journal* is published quarterly when possible. The following is a list of Cancer Victors and Friends chapters and phone numbers. Chapters usually publish their own newsletters. Contact international headquarters for exact addresses.

California
Playa del Rey: (310) 822-5032
Santa Barbara: (805) 969-9157
San Jose: (408) 269-7466

Florida
Fort Lauderdale: (305) 733-9121, 946-2770
Miami: (305) 796-3549
Orlando: (407) 859-1931
West Palm Beach: (407) 798-4536,
969-2810

Georgia
Atlanta: (404) 634-4101, 426-4399

Illinois
Cicero: (708) 780-6188
Niles: (708) 692-2596

New Jersey
Matawan: (201) 583-1274

New York
Hicksville: (516) 796-3964

Washington
Bothell: (206) 481-4351

Australia
Melbourne: 011-61-03-836-8764

Canada
Victoria: (604) 360-2988

Illness Addressed

Cancer.

Type of Information Offered

Reports and information on alternative therapies and recent cancer studies.

Costs

Membership (yearly): $25. Sustaining member: $100. Life member: $300. Perpetual member: $1,000. Membership and donations are tax-deductible.

International Health Information Institute

3231 Lowry Road
Los Angeles, California 90027-2206
United States

(213) 664-0714
Fax: (213) 664-3214

Contact Person

Jack Tropp.

Primary Personnel

Jack Tropp, Ph.D., director.

Directions

Available on request.

Background

Jack Tropp, a freelance writer, lecturer, and consultant for more than thirty-five years, has been investigating and reporting on health and nutrition, with a focus on holistic approaches to the treatment of cancer. He was Japan correspondent for *Prevention Magazine;* research director of Shangri-La Natural Hygiene Institute in Florida; director of Cancer Resource Center in Los Angeles; and information and education director of Valley Cancer Institute in Panorama City, California. He received the Bronze Halo Award from the Southern California Motion Picture Council for his book *Cancer: A Healing Crisis—The Whole-Body Approach to Cancer Therapy.* The council cited the book as an "outstanding contribution to humanity."

Illness Addressed

Cancer.

Type of Information Offered

This service provides options, insights, and connections with physicians, holistic practitioners, clinics, and hospitals around the world to help sort out today's often confusing collection of alternative/holistic treatments. The institute does not diagnose, prescribe, or treat, but offers information and guidance to assist the client with choices relative to the particular cancer problem. It is sometimes possible, even at the first telephone consultation, to provide a highly-focused protocol to the inquiring patient, family member, or friend. By following through with the physicians, clinics, and hospitals suggested, the patient is then able to gather the precise additional information needed. The institute's experience indicates that in many cases, just the first discussion (and the resulting contacts) has significantly helped to clarify confusing factors for the patient. This allows the patient to reach a decision regarding a plan of action, with confidence that it will be the most promising course of action available.

Related Readings

Provided as requested by the individual patient.

Costs

$50 per consultation. If any additional research and reporting is necessary, charges will be based on a case-by-case situation.

Method of Payment

Personal checks, traveler's checks, and money orders are accepted.

International Holistic Center Inc.

1042 Willow Creek Road A111-151
Prescott, Arizona 86301
United States

(520) 771-1742

Contact Person

Stan Kalson, director.

Background

This organization provides information and referrals concerning holistic health care in Arizona and beyond.

Illness Addressed

A wellness approach to prevent illness.

Type of Information Offered

The center provides information about holistic health care and helps publish the *Holistic H.E.L.P. Handbook.* It offers massages, a support group, networking activities, information and referral services, and a speaker's bureau.

Related Readings

Holistic H.E.L.P. Handbook by Stan Kalson.

Holistic H.E.L.P. Directory. This directory has two editions. The Greater Phoenix edition covers Phoenix, Scottsdale, Tempe, Mesa, and Glendale; and the Northern Arizona edition covers Prescott, Sedona, Cottonwood, and Flagstaff.

Costs

$10 for the handbook, $2 for each directory.

Mankind Research Foundation

1315 Apple Avenue
Silver Spring, Maryland 20910
United States

(301) 587-8686

Contact Person

Dr. Carl Schleicher.

Primary Personnel

T. Gooden, M.D.; A. Onyegbula, M.D.

Directions

Near I-95 and I-496 intersection.

Background

The foundaton has been active in alternative medicine since 1972. It produces a number of products in this area, and also operates alternative medical clinics to make available alternative medical treatments.

Illness Addressed

Cancer, multiple sclerosis, amyotrophic lateral sclerosis, viral blood infections including HIV/AIDS and hepatitis, and neuromuscular disorders.

Type of Information Offered

Descriptive flyers on services; clinical results of therapies offered.

Related Readings

Into the Light by W.C. Douglas, M.D.
Biofeedback by Dr. Barbara Brown.

Costs

The foundation's fees are nominal, since it is a nonprofit group with low overhead, and uses volunteers where possible.

Method of Payment

Cash, checks, Visa, and MasterCard are accepted, as well as insurance and Medicare.

National Health Federation

212 West Foothill Boulevard
P.O. Box 688
Monrovia, California 91016
United States

(818) 357-2181
(818) 359-8334
Fax: (818) 303-0642

Primary Personnel

Patrick Van Mauck, chairman of the board; Dr. Jonathan Wright, M.D., president; Maureen Salaman, vice president.

Background

National Health Federation is a nonprofit consumer-oriented organization devoted exclusively to health matters. It is dedicated to preserving freedom of choice in health care issues—not only in the prevention of disease, but in the promotion of wellness. There are 108 active chapters around the country; for a listing, please write or call the Monrovia headquarters. The federation has a lobbyist in Washington D.C. to defend health rights.

Illness Addressed

Cancer and other health problems.

Type of Information Offered

National Health Federation offers conventions, seminars, and a monthly news journal for members. Last year, conventions were held in Pasadena, California; Chicago (Rosemont), Illinois; Pittsburgh, Pennsylvania; Denver, Colorado; and Orlando, Florida.

Costs

$36 for a regular membership. $1,000 for life membership. $2,000 for perpetual membership.

Method of Payment

Checks or credit cards are accepted.

National Self-Help Clearinghouse

25 West 43rd Street
Room 620
New York, New York 10036
United States

Primary Personnel

Frank Riessman, director; Audrey Gartner, executive director.

Background

The National Self-Help Clearinghouse was founded in 1976 to facilitate access to self-help groups and to increase awareness of the importance of mutual support groups. Self-help group members feel less isolated knowing others share similar problems; they exchange ideas and methods for handling problems; they actively work on their attitude and behavior to make positive changes in their lives; and they gain a sense of control over their own lives, leaving them less overwhelmed by their problems.

Illness Addressed

The whole range of life's crises.

Type of Information Offered

For a list of local self-help clearinghouses throughout the United States, or for information about the location of a specific self-help group, just send in your inquiry along with a stamped, self-addressed envelope.

Costs

Publications are sold; inquiries are answered for free. *Self-Help Reporter,* one-year subscription (four issues): $10. *How to Organize a Self-Help Group:* $6. *Organizing a Self-Help Clearinghouse:* $5.

Method of Payment

Personal checks are accepted.

Nutrition Education Association Inc.

3647 Glen Haven
Houston, Texas 77025
United States

(713) 665-2946

P.O. Box 20301
Houston, Texas 77225
United States

Contact Person

Bill Long, secretary.

Primary Personnel

Ruth Yale Long, Ph.D., nutritionist.

Directions

Two miles west of medical center.

Background

Nutrition Education Association is a nonprofit organization dedicated to educating the public about the importance of good nutrition for their health.

Illness Addressed

Cancer and various degenerative diseases.

Type of Information Offered

Nutrition education through books.

Related Readings

Crackdown on Cancer With Good Nutrition by Ruth Yale Long. Nutrition Education Association, 1983. Second edition 1989.

Home Study Course in the New Nutrition by Ruth Yale Long.

Switchover! The Anti-Cancer Cooking Plan for Today's Parents and Their Children by Ruth Yale Long.

These books are available through mail order.

Also recommended are books on nutrition by Jeffrey Bland, Linus Pauling, Roger Williams, and Emanuel Cheraskin.

Costs

Contact the Nutrition Education Association for a complete list of available books and their prices.

Method of Payment

Personal checks are accepted.

Patient Advocates for Advanced Cancer Treatments Inc. (PAACT)

1143 Parmelee N.W.
Grand Rapids, Michigan 49504
United States

(616) 453-1477
Fax: (616) 453-1846

Contact Person

Lloyd J. Ney, president.

Background

PAACT claims to be the largest organization of its kind in the world, with more than 23,000 patients and more than 800 physicians of various disciplines counted among its members. PAACT's prostate cancer oncology group is a privately funded, cooperative research organization that investigates prostate cancer and its treatments.

Illness Addressed

Prostate cancer.

Type of Information Offered

State-of-the-art detection, diagnostics, evaluation, and treatments for all stages of prostate cancer and for related problems.

Related Readings

Onco-Logic (newsletter for physicians only).

Prostate Cancer Review.

Cancer Communication Newsletter.

"The Gland Illusion" in *American Health Magazine.* December 1990.

Costs

Voluntary donation and/or PAACT membership, which starts at $25.

Patient Rights Legal Action Fund

202 West 78th Street—3E
New York, New York 10024
United States

Primary Personnel

Avis Lang, coordinator.

Background

The Patient Rights Legal Action Fund was initially formed in August 1985, in response to what it deemed government violations of the basic constitutional rights of the cancer patients of Stanislaw R. Burzynski, M.D., Ph.D. It organized a class-action lawsuit to help ensure uninterrupted patient access to the clinic, stressing the return of past and present patients' medical records and insurance and billing files seized by the United States Food and Drug Administration in July 1985. Although the patients' case was largely dismissed and the United States Supreme Court declined to hear an appeal of the dismissal, the case succeeded in becoming a focal point for educating the public about the problems of both doctors and patients who use nonstandard cancer therapies.

Related Readings

A booklet of excerpts from the 1,800-page official transcript of the October 1985 court hearing, including an introduction and explanatory notes. It is called *On the Public Record: Cancer Patients Take the United States Government to Court.*

A one-hour videotape, *Cancer Scandal: The Policies and Politics of Failure,* is also available. In the tape, three well-known science writers—Robert G. Houston, Patrick M.

McGrady Jr., and Ralph W. Moss—explore the nature of the cancer industry in a no-holds-barred roundtable discussion. Also available is a lengthy interview with Stanislaw R. Burzynski, M.D., Ph.D., "The Disease of Information Processing."

Costs

The booklet costs $7.50, plus $1.50 postage and handling. The VHS videotape costs $29.95 plus $3 postage and handling. The interview, as well as other articles and information, is available on request, preferably accompanied by a stamped, self-addressed envelope.

Method of Payment

Checks drawn on United States banks and postal money orders in United States dollars are accepted. Make payable to IFCO-PRLAF. All contributions are tax-deductible.

Patient-Directed Consultations

4637 Ulloa Street
San Francisco, California 94116
United States

(415) 681-5357
Fax: (415) 681-9734
E-mail: renneker@well.com

Primary Personnel

Mark Renneker, M.D., a board-certified, university-affiliated family physician.

Background

Patient-Directed Consultations provides help to patients who can't seem to find the help or information they need, or who feel they have too much information and too many options, yet still need to make a decision about what to do next. Dr. Renneker becomes a patient's own medical consultant, researcher, and advocate, working to help the patient (and family members, as designated) gain the information, understanding, and authority to move forward. This sometimes entails helping to resolve conflicts that patients and family members may have with their practitioners or the present care plan. He practices what he calls "optimistic medicine"—no matter how desperate or hopeless a situation may appear, there are always new things to try. He does not assume care for the patient, nor provide treatment, but he does help find and arrange the best possible treatments, drawing on the full range of conventional, experimental, and alternative therapies.

Illness Addressed

Dr. Renneker is happy to consider helping any person (or family), regardless of where they live or their medical problem.

Type of Information Offered

First, a comprehensive write-up about the practice is sent. This includes a questionnaire to fill in and return for Dr. Renneker's review, to see if he feels he can help. In the majority of cases, an initial phone consultation is then arranged. At that time, the situation is discussed in depth, and a plan is made as to how best to proceed. This often involves further review of the complete medical record and—with the patient's permission—discussing the case with the treating practitioners. Comprehensive computer- and library-based research is usually then pursued, which Dr. Renneker analyzes, annotates, and organizes into a workbook, which is sent to and then discussed with the patient and family. This often leads to a deeper level of research, involving Dr. Renneker's calling specialists (traditional and alternative) around the world, seeking clinical and pre-publication research information, as well as their expert opinions (and help) on the case. Dr. Renneker communicates with the patient and family each step of the way, assisting in decision-making and case-planning as needed. He accepts no more than one new patient per week, allowing him to spend as much time as needed on every case.

Related Readings

A comprehensive write-up is available from Dr. Renneker's office, which describes the range and types of cases he works with, his background and publications, how he works and charges, and how to arrange for his services.

Costs

The write-up and questionnaire are free (and sometimes help a person realize how to resolve the problem on his or her own). The initial sixty- to seventy-five minute phone consultation is $250. Thereafter, a sliding scale is used, ranging from $50 to $300 per hour.

People Against Cancer

604 East Street
Otho, Iowa 50569-0010
United States

(515) 972-4444

Primary Personnel

Frank Wiewel, executive director and founder; Marie Dallman, volunteer; Denise Wiewel, volunteer; Charlotte Christie, volunteer.

Background

People Against Cancer is a nonprofit grassroots organization whose mission is to make deep inroads into the cancer problem by encouraging the development of innovative approaches and seeking new directions in the war on cancer. It works toward preserving, protecting, and enhancing medical freedom of choice. It promotes a pollution-free environment. Members include people with cancer, their loved ones, and others who are concerned with making rapid progress against the disease.

Illness Addressed

Cancer.

Type of Information Offered

People Against Cancer has developed a new program for people with cancer called the Alternative Therapy Program. The goal of this program is to provide options for people with cancer, and to answer the complex questions about treatment alternatives, such as what therapy might be best, and what approach might offer the best chances for survival and quality of life. The organization feels it is important to understand all options, from conventional to alternative, in order for people to make truly informed decisions about treatment. It believes that people with cancer have very fundamental rights—the right to know and the right to choose. People Against Cancer publishes and distributes books and other materials on innovative approaches to cancer prevention and treatment, counsels members, holds public and professional seminars, addresses political issues, provides information on the role of diet and nutrition in cancer, helps people form self-help and empowerment groups, teaches grassroots-organizing techniques, and arranges for members to receive discounts on medical-related travel costs.

Related Readings

Options: Revolutionary Ideas in the War on Cancer, a bimonthly newsletter.

Costs

Annual memberships cost $25 (regular), $50 (contributing), $100 (sustaining), $250 (supporting), and $500 (benefactor). The higher the level of membership, the more free books and services the member receives. Membership fees and donations are tax-deductible.

Method of Payment

Checks, Visa, and MasterCard are accepted.

Planetree Health Resource Center

2040 Webster Street
San Francisco, California 94115
United States

(415) 923-3680

Primary Personnel

Tracey Cosgrove, M.L.I.S.

Background

Planetree is a nonprofit consumer health library dedicated to helping patients and consumers become active participants in their own health and medical care. Planetree was founded in 1978 by a group of consumer advocates, educators, physicians, and business and cultural leaders.

Illness Addressed

Cancer and all medical conditions.

Type of Information Offered

A range of health and medical information—from lay-oriented publications to the latest professional literature to an extensive collection of alternative or complementary therapy books and journal articles. Planetree offers people who are unable to visit the library the following services:

Computer searched bibliography. Planetree will search the databases of the National Library of Medicine to produce a bibliography of up to forty article citations. Citations include the available title, author, author address, source, and summaries of articles.

PDQ computer search. Sponsored by the National Cancer Institute, this database produces concise and current information on specific cancer diagnoses in a report format. Planetree provides both the "Information for Patients" and "State-of-the-Art Information" sections and details on prognosis, staging, and standard and investigational treatment protocols being conducted in the United States.

In-depth information packet. This is an individualized comprehensive selection of the current medical and lay literature on a diagnosis or topic, with particular emphasis on the patient's focus of interest (e.g., complementary therapies). The packet is usually fifty to sixty pages in length; and may include: selections from current medical textbooks, journals, and consumer health literature; materials describing complementary treatment options; a current computer search from medical literature databases; and the names and addresses of national and local organizations, support groups, or contact people dedicated to sharing information on your topic.

Costs

People who visit the library have access to information at no cost. People who cannot get to the library will be charged the following fees: computer searched bibliography: $35; PDQ computer search: $25; in-depth information packet: $100.

Method of Payment

Cash, checks, money orders, Visa, and MasterCard are accepted.

Private Cancer Clinic Tours

P.O. Box 530218
San Diego, California 92153
United States

(619) 475-3834

Contact Person

Roberto Rodriguez.

Directions

Clients are picked up at Americana Inn and Suites, 815 W. San Ysidro Boulevard, San Ysidro, California 92173, (800) 553-3933.

Illness Addressed

Cancer and immune deficiency disorders.

Type of Information Offered

Personalized tours of the various clinics in Tijuana, Mexico, are available any day of the week with advanced notice. If possible, patients should bring test results or health information documentation. Some of the clinics will have doctors available to make preliminary suggestions on cases. Patients should also bring a tape recorder or writing tablet to record information. For those wishing to spend the night, special lodging rates are available by contacting Americana Inn and Suites directly. Cars may be parked at Americana Inn and Suites during the tour. For those arriving the day before the tour and spending the night, doctors from the various clinics may be available to give complimentary information sessions at the Americana Inn and Suites conference room (advanced notice required). The tour's pickup time is 9:30 a.m., and the length of the tour depends upon the number of clinics visited and the length of stay at each clinic.

Costs

$75.00 per person for groups of two or more, $125 for one person, up to eight hours in Mexico visiting the clinics.

Method of Payment

Checks, cash, or money orders are accepted.

Tour of Tijuana, Mexico Clinics

P.O. Box 4651
Modesto, California 95352-4651
United States

(209) 529-4697

Contact Person

Frank or Rosario Cousineau.

Background

The Cancer Control Society and Life Support sponsor this one-day tour approximately six times per year. Custom or specialized tours are available upon request. California nurses may take the tour for ten C.E. units.

Illness Addressed

Cancer, arthritis, multiple sclerosis, and others.

Type of Information Offered

Guided tour of alternative therapy clinics in Tijuana, Mexico. The tour visits the following alternative therapy clinics: American Biologics, American Metabolic Institute, Bio-Medical Center, Genesis West Clinic, Gerson Institute, Oasis Hospital, Hospital Santa Monica, and Stella Maris. Lectures are given at many of the clinics. Departure and return times are as follows: Pasadena Hilton, 150 S. Los Robles Avenue, Pasadena: depart 7:00 a.m., return 11:30 p.m. Grand Hotel, 7 Freedman Way, Anaheim (Orange County): depart 7:45 a.m., return 11:00 p.m. Visitors Information Center, 2688 E. Mission Bay Drive, San Diego: depart 9:15 a.m., return 9:00 p.m. Tourist Information (across the border), Tijuana, Mexico: depart 9:45 a.m., return 8:30 p.m.

Costs

The cost of the tour is $75 (tax-deductible) per person, regardless of pickup point.

Lunch will be provided at one of the clinics, and snacks will be served en route and at the other clinics. California nurses taking the tour for C.E. credits pay $100.

Method of Payment

Send check or money order at least seven days in advance, or call to make arrangements to pay upon boarding bus.

World Research Foundation

Product Fullfillmet:
41 Bell Rock Plaza, Suite C
Sedona, Arizona 86351
United States

(520) 284-3300
Fax: (520) 284-3530

Executive Offices:
20501 Ventura Boulevard, Suite 100
Woodland Hills, California 91364

(818) 999-5483
Fax: (818) 227-6484

Contact Person

Adele Ross.

Primary Personnel

LaVerne Ross and Steven Ross, cofounders.

Background

Founded in 1984, World Research Foundation is a nonprofit health and environmental information network. It includes five offices worldwide and an extensive library system containing books dating to the 1600s in English and 200 B.C. in other languages. The foundation is linked to more than 500 computer databases that provide access to important medical, scientific, and environmental information from more than 100 countries. The primary purpose of the organization is to locate, gather, codify, classify, and disseminate all available information dealing with health (both traditional and nontraditional, from ancient times to the present) and the environment. World Research Foundation's services are available to the public, health professionals, and the news media. The foundation acts as a consultant to governmental agencies. The foundation's research libraries are open to the public.

Illness Addressed

All illnesses.

Type of Information Offered

Two different types of health information files are available. A library search packet contains complementary, alternative, and nontraditional therapies gathered from books, periodicals, and other forms of literature. A computer search packet contains the most up-to-date allopathic (i.e., pharmaceutical and surgical) information, which tends to be very technical and uses medical terminology. The data is gathered from 5,000 medical journals worldwide and includes the latest forty to fifty abstracted articles (when available).

Related Readings

World Research News, a quarterly newsletter, contains worldwide health information. $20 per year in the United States or $25 per year for an international subscription. Also available are books, audio tapes, and videotapes on numerous health topics.

Costs

Library search packet: $60 (California residents add sales tax). Computer search packet: $60 (California residents add sales tax). All donations are appreciated and are tax-deductible. For a $40 donation, you receive discounts on World Research Foundation health congresses, books, videotapes, and audio tapes, plus a subscription to the foundation's quarterly newsletter. For one dollar, you will receive a brochure on the foundation, a sample issue of *World Research News,* and a listing of available books, audio tapes, and videotapes.

Method of Payment

Checks, money orders, Visa, and MasterCard are accepted.

INFORMATION SERVICES

Overseas (Australia, Netherlands, United Kingdom)

Cancer Information & Support Society

1/51 Crown Road
Queenscliff 2096
New South Wales
Australia

Contact Person

Secretary.

Primary Personnel

Donald J. Benjamin.

Background

The society, a nonprofit organization, was established in 1981 to provide people with information on holistic, nonaggressive, low-toxic methods of overcoming disease.

Illness Addressed

Cancer and other degenerative diseases.

Type of Information Offered

A library, videos, tapes, research papers, information on overseas clinics, and other materials are available in the office. Office hours are 10:00 a.m. to 1:00 p.m. and 2:00 p.m. to 4:30 p.m. Wednesdays.

Related Readings

The society publishes a bimonthly newsletter and the *Cancer Information & Support Society Handbook*.

Costs

$25 for a one-year membership, which includes a subscription to the society's newsletter.

Moerman Vereniging

Postbus 14
6674 ZG Herveld
Netherlands

011-31-488-451221
Fax: 011-31-488-45812

Contact Person

Doctors should contact Albert Ronhaar, M.D., Parallelweg 60, 7782 PH De Krim, or by telephone: 011-310-524-571210. Patients have a different contact and should telephone 011-310-689-98350.

Background

Only a few countries in Europe have Moerman doctors. The doctors prevent and combat cancer by having the patient take certain vitamins and minerals and adopt a particular diet and lifestyle. Members of Moerman Vereniging are cancer victims treated by the therapy of Dr. Moerman. Some people who sympathize but are not cancer victims have also joined. The organization supports patients and people who have no cancer but believe in this method. A list of doctors who can give this treatment is available.

Illness Addressed

Degenerative diseases, primarily cancer.

Type of Information Offered

New patients who call Moerman Vereniging speak to a volunteer, who supplies information about the therapy and the Moerman Vereniging, and the address and phone number of a Moerman doctor who can accept the patient very soon for a short visit (about one hour). The volunteer also supplies the phone number of a person who has recovered from the same kind of cancer, and the phone number of a nearby person who can accompany the patient to the doctor. The patient receives a magazine and diet list, which he or she can start following even before visiting the doctor. The diet allows many foods (such as buttermilk, brown rice, cooked and raw vegetables, pea soup, whole wheat bread, and almost all fruits), disallows many foods (such as meat, fish, poultry, coffee, tea, white flour products, and yogurt), and makes lifestyle suggestions (such as no drinking of alcoholic beverages, no smoking, no sunbathing, and no second hand smoke). The vitamins and minerals involved in the treatment are usually taken orally and require the doctor's prescription. Patients stay at their own homes and see their Moerman doctor once month.

Related Readings

Dr. Moerman's Anti-Cancer Diet: Holland's Revolutionary Nutritional Program for Combatting Cancer by Ruth Jochems. Avery Publishing Group, 1990.
A Solution to the Cancer Problem by C. Moerman. Moerman Vereniging.

Costs

Staff volunteers do not receive fees. The estimated fees of the doctor and chemist were not submitted for publication.

New Approaches to Cancer

5, Larksfield, Egham
Surrey, TW20 0RB
England
United Kingdom

011-0784-433610

Primary Personnel

Colin Ryder Richardson.

Background

New Approaches to Cancer, a registered charity, considers its holistic program to be a complement to the treatment of cancer as offered by the conventional medical profession. New Approaches acts as the nerve center of a network throughout the United Kingdom to promote research, organize workshops and conferences to improve attitudes, and show that cancer can be prevented and overcome. It does not have its own clinic, but it does have 450 associates around the United Kingdom, ranging from individual therapists to support groups and residential clinics. It promotes the benefits of holistic and self-help methods of healing for those with cancer.

Illness Addressed

Cancer.

Type of Information Offered

Nonmedical advice on the holistic approach to cancer.

Related Readings

The Holistic Approach to Cancer by Dr. Ian Pearce.
New Approaches to Cancer by Shirley Harrison.
The Bristol Programme by Penny Brohn.
Raw Energy by Leslie and Susannah Kenton.
How to Meditate by Dr. Lawrence LeShan.
Cancer as a Turning Point by Dr. Lawrence LeShan.
The Wealth Within by Dr. Ainslie Meares.
The Miracle of Colour Healing by Vicky Wall.
You Can Heal Your Life by Louise L. Hay. Coleman, 1985.
Emma Says Goodbye by Carolyn Nystrom.
Love, Medicine and Miracles by Dr. Bernie Siegel. Harper & Row, 1986.

Peace, Love and Healing by Dr. Bernie Siegel.

Getting Well Again by O. Carl Simonton, Stephanie Matthews-Simonton, and James Creighton. J.P. Tarcher, 1978.

Mind Over Cancer by Colin Ryder Richardson.

Costs

New Approaches to Cancer is a national registered charity. All work is offered without charge, but donations are accepted.

A Region-by-Region Look at Treatment Centers, Educational Centers, Support Programs, and Information Services

This region-by-region listing will help you locate those centers, services, and programs that can be found in your area. Each of these resources is discussed in detail in this book. The code letter following the entry will direct you to the section of the text containing complete information: **T**=Treatment Centers; **E**=Educational Centers; **S**=Support Programs; **I**=Information Services.

AUSTRALIA
(I.J.) Bullen **(E)**
Cancer Information & Support Society **(I)**
Cancer Support Association Inc. **(S)**
The Gawler Foundation **(E)**
Hippocrates Health Centre of Australia **(E)**
Relaxation Centre of Queensland, Limited **(S)**

BAHAMAS
Immuno-Augmentative Therapy Centre **(T)**

CANADA
Cancer Counselling Center **(S)**
Cose Inc. **(T)**

HOPE Cancer Health Society **(S)**
Northern Health Inc. **(T)**
Pacific Center for Naturopathic Medicine **(T)**
Schafer's Health Centre Ltd. **(T)**

CUBA
Ozone Research Center **(T)**

ENGLAND
The Bristol Cancer Help Centre **(T)**
The Hale Clinic **(E)**
Hereford Cancer Help Clinic **(S)**
New Approaches to Cancer **(I)**
Park Attwood Clinic **(T)**
Plymouth Natural Health and Healing

Centre **(S)**
Thorpe Bay Self-Help Cancer Group **(S)**

GERMANY
(Hartmut) Baltin, M.D. **(T)**
Bio Med Klinik **(T)**
Hufeland Klinik for Holistic
  Immunotherapy **(T)**
Institute for Immunology and Thymus
  Research **(T)**
(Dr. Helmut) Keller **(T)**
(Hans A.) Nieper, M.D. **(T)**

HONG KONG
Optimum Health Centre **(T)**

IRELAND
The East Clinic **(T)**

ISRAEL
(Joseph) Brenner, M.D. **(T)**

JAPAN
Holistic Keihoku Hospital **(T)**
Hotaka Yojoen Holistic Health Center **(E)**

MEXICO
Advanced Medical Group **(T)**
The Alivizatos Treatment—Hospital
  American Biologics **(T)**
American Metabolic Institute **(T)**
American Biologics-Mexico S.A. Medical
  Center **(T)**
Bio-Medical Center **(T)**
Center for General Medicine and
  Acupuncture **(T)**
Centro Profesional Unidad de
  Neurodiagnostico **(T)**
(Ernesto) Contreras Jr., M.D. **(T)**
Cydel Medical Center **(T)**

Europa Institute of Integrated Medicine **(T)**
GenesisWest Research Institute for
  Biological Medicine **(T)**
Gerson Institute (Hospital Meridien de
  Playas de Tijuana) **(T)**
Gerson Research Organization/CHIPSA
  (T)
Hospital Bajanor S.A. de C.V. **(T)**
Hospital Santa Monica **(T)**
Institute of Chronic Disease **(T)**
Instituto Cientifico de Regeneracion, S.A.
  (T)
International Center for Medical and
  Biological Research, Inc. **(T)**
International Medical Center **(T)**
The Kuhnau Center **(T)**
Mission Medical Clinic **(T)**
Oasis Hospital **(T)**
Program for Studies of Alternative
  Medicines **(T)**
St. Joesph Medical Center **(T)**
Sierra Clinic Inc. **(T)**
Stella Maris Clinic **(T)**

NETHERLANDS
Moerman Vereniging **(I)**

NEW ZEALAND
Bay of Plenty Environmental Health
  Clinic **(T)**
Medical Research Inc. **(E)**

PHILIPPINES
Bio Medical Health Center **(T)**

PORTUGAL
Health Center of Lisbon **(T)**

SPAIN
(J. Buxalleu) Font **(T)**

SWITZERLAND
Paracelsus Klinik **(T)**

UNITED STATES
North Central
(Vahagn) Agbabian, D.O. **(T)**
Block Medical Center **(T)**
(Brian E.) Briggs, M.D. **(T)**
Cancer Counseling Center **(S)**
Cancer Prevention Coalition **(I)**
Cancer Treatment Centers of America **(T)**
Center for the Improvement of Human Functioning International, Inc. **(E)**
Creative Health Institute **(E)**
(Ross A.) Hauser, M.D., D.C. **(T)**
Health, Research, and Referral Center **(I)**
(Edward W.) McDonagh, D.O.; (Charles J.) Rudolph, D.O., Ph.D. **(T)**
Natural Medicine Clinic **(T)**
Partners in Wellness **(T)**
Patient Advocates for Advanced Cancer Treatments Inc. (PAACT) **(I)**
People Against Cancer **(I)**
Shealy Institute for Comprehensive Health Care **(T)**
(Georg F.) Springer, M.D. **(T)**
Waisbren Clinic **(T)**
Wellness House **(S)**

Northeast
(Jan) Abruzzo **(S)**
The Ash Center for Comprehensive Medicine **(T)**
Atkins Center for Complementary Medicine **(T)**
(Pearl) Bennette-Atkin, R.N., M.A., C.S. **(E)**
(Ruth) Bolletino, Ph.D. **(S)**
Center for Advancement in Cancer Education **(I)**
Center for Nutrition and Preventive Medicine **(T)**
Center for Preventive Medicine and Homeopathy **(T)**
The Centers for Progressive Medicine **(T)**
Consciousness Research and Training Project Inc. **(S)**
Exceptional Cancer Patients (ECaP) **(S)**
Foundation for Advancement in Cancer Therapy (FACT) **(I)**
Foundation for Cartilage and Immunology Research **(T)**
(Nicholas) Gonzalez, M.D. **(T)**
(Dayton) Haigney, M.D. **(T)**
Healing Choices Cancer Report Service **(I)**
Health Achievement Center **(T)**
Health Quest Clinic **(T)**
The Hoffman Center **(T)**
(P.) Jayalakshmi, M.D. **(T)**
(Roy E.) Kerry, M.D. **(T)**
Kushi Institute **(E)**
(Lawrence) LeShan, Ph.D. **(S)**
Magaziner Medical Center **(T)**
Mantell Medical Clinic **(T)**
Metabolic Associates **(T)**
National Self-Help Clearinghouse **(I)**
New Life Health Center **(E)**
Patient Rights Legal Action Fund **(I)**
Revici Life Science Center **(T)**
(Michael B.) Schacter, M.D., P.C., and Associates **(T)**
(Ron) Schmid, N.D. **(T)**
(Charles) Simone, M.D. **(T)**
Syracuse Cancer Research Institute, Inc. **(E)**
Wellspring Foundation of New England, Inc. **(S)**
Woodlands Medical Center, Inc. **(T)**
Writers and Research, Inc. **(E)**
(S.) Yurkovsky, M.D. **(T)**
(Victoria) Zupa, N.D. **(T)**

South
Accent on Health **(T)**

Advanced Medical Group **(T)**
Arlin J. Brown Information Center Inc. **(I)**
(Paul V.) Beals, M.D. **(T)**
Burzynski Clinic **(T)**
Cancer Treatment Centers of America **(T)**
Carolina Center for Bio-Oxidative
Medicine **(T)**
Carolina Health Quest **(T)**
Center for Metabolic Disorders **(T)**
Center for Science in the Public Interest **(I)**
(Elisabeth Anne) Cole, M.D. **(T)**
Cypress Consultants **(I)**
Environmental and Preventive Health
Center of Atlanta **(T)**
Florida Preventive Health Services,
Inc. **(T)**
The Georgia CancerHelp Program **(S)**
The Health Resource, Inc. **(I)**
Hippocrates Health Institute **(E)**
International Academy of Nutrition
and Preventive Medicine **(I)**
Life Extension Nutrition Center **(E)**
Lost Horizon Health Awareness Center **(T)**
Mankind Research Foundation **(I)**
(Thomas) McNaughton, M.D. **(T)**
New Hope Medical Center **(T)**
Nutrition Education Association Inc. **(I)**
Panama City Clinic **(T)**
Perlmutter Health Center **(T)**
(William H.) Philpott, M.D. **(T)**
(Vladimir) Rizov, M.D. **(T)**
The Ruscombe Mansion Community
Health Center **(T)**
The Rushing Clinic, P.A. **(T)**
(Ahmad) Shamim, M.D. **(T)**
Smith Farm **(S)**
Southeast Research Foundation Inc. **(E)**
(Colin) Tipping, M.Ed., Dip.H. **(S)**
Warren's Clinic **(T)**
(Ray) Wunderlich Jr., M.D. **(T)**

West
Advanced Medical Clinic **(T)**
AeroStat Air & Land Ambulance, Inc. **(S)**
Alternative Medicine Associates **(T)**
Alternative Medicine Center of
Colorado **(T)**
The American Health Institute, Inc. **(S)**
(Scott V.) Anderson, M.D., D.C. **(T)**
(Daniel) Beilin, O.M.D., L.Ac. **(T)**
Bio Medical Health Center **(T)**
Bio-Ethics Medical Center, Inc. **(T)**
The Bresler Center, Inc. **(S)**
(W. Douglas) Brodie, M.D. **(T)**
Buchholz Medical Group **(T)**
Burzynski Patients Organization **(S)**
Cancer Control Society and Cancer
Book House **(I)**
Cancer Support and Education Center **(S)**
Cancer Support Community **(S)**
CanHelp **(I)**
(Richard) Casdorph, M.D. **(T)**
Center for Attitudinal Healing **(S)**
Central Coast Holistic Medical Services
(T)
The Chopra Center for Well Being **(E)**
Colorado Outward Bound School **(S)**
Committee for Freedom of Choice in
Medicine Inc. **(I)**
Commonweal Cancer Help Program **(S)**
(Dale) Figtree, Ph.D. **(E)**
George Ohsawa Macrobiotic
Foundation **(E)**
Gerson Healing Centers of America **(T)**
Gerson Therapy Self-Help **(E)**
Harmony Hill of Union **(S)**
Healing Alternatives Network **(I)**
Health Action **(E)**
HealthQuarters Lodge **(E)**
Holistic Medical Center **(T)**
(Richard P.) Huemer, M.D. **(T)**

Hydeout **(E)**

International Association of Cancer Victors and Friends **(I)**

International Health Information Institute **(I)**

International Holistic Center Inc. **(I)**

The Intimacy and Healing Project **(S)**

Izaac David Frees Organic Health Research **(E)**

(Richard A.) Kunin, M.D. **(T)**

Linus Pauling Institute **(E)**

Livingston Foundation Medical Center **(T)**

The McDougall Program at St. Helena Hospital **(T)**

Medical Health and Fitness **(E)**

Mind/Body Center **(S)**

(Robert) Nagourney, M.D. **(T)**

National Health Federation **(I)**

Nevada Clinic **(T)**

O Ka Mana Ka Ho'ola **(S)**

Optimum Health Institute of San Diego **(E)**

Pacific Center for Naturopathic Medicine **(T)**

Patient-Directed Consultations **(I)**

(Ray) Peat, Ph.D. **(E)**

Planetree Health Resource Center **(I)**

Preventive Medical Center of Marin, Inc. **(T)**

Private Cancer Clinic Tours **(I)**

(James R.) Privitera, M.D. **(T)**

Psychosomatics **(S)**

Resources for Wholeness and Achievement **(S)**

Rosabell Medical Group **(T)**

(Robert) Rowen, M.D. **(T)**

Simonton Cancer Center **(S)**

(Suzanne) Skinner, Ph.D. **(T)**

(Leila) Stephens **(S)**

Synergy Seminars **(S)**

Tour of Tijuana, Mexico Clinics **(I)**

Valley Cancer Institute **(T)**

(Virginia) Veach, Ph.D., M.F.C.C., P.T. **(S)**

Vega Study Center **(E)**

Vital-Life Institute **(T)**

Well Being International Inc. **(S)**

Wellness Center Associates, Inc. **(E)**

The Wellness Community **(S)**

(Julian) Whitaker, M.D. **(T)**

World Research Foundation **(I)**

Glossary

Some of the terms that appear throughout this book may be unfamiliar to you. Although a number of these terms can be found in a standard medical dictionary, many are used strictly in the field of alternative therapy. This glossary defines those terms that are part of the vocabulary of alternative therapy—and even defines some terms that do not appear in this book. In addition, it defines many of the abbreviations that are used in these listings and in other literature on this subject.

Acupuncture is based on the theory that energy flows along specific pathways or "meridians" connecting the organs deep in the body with the acupoints on the surface of the body. In diseased conditions, there is a breakdown of the free flow of energy. By piercing the skin at certain points, the energy flow is stimulated or sedated so as to restore the functioning equilibrium.

AMID (Arthur morphologic immuno-status differential) is a microscopic examination of leukocytes (white blood cells) from specially prepared and stained thin blood films.

Amino acid therapy consists of infusions of protein to restore the body to a more natural condition. It is used in some metabolic cancer programs.

Amygdalin. *See* Laetrile.

Anabolic compounds allow the conversion of nutritive material into complex living matter in the constructive metabolism.

Anthroposophical medicine, developed by Rudolph Steiner, is a method of treating the whole body by addressing spiritual as well as physical aspects. Medications including mistletoe (*Viscum album*) as well as a special diet, color therapy, artistic therapy, curative eurythmy (movement), and specially prepared baths are included. It is widely available in special hospitals and clinics found mostly in Germany and Switzerland.

Antineoplastons, according to Dr. Stanislaw Burzynski, are a class of compounds produced by the living organism to protect it against neoplastic (tumorous) growth through a non-immunological process that does not significantly inhibit the growth of normal tissue.

Autogenous vaccine is a vaccine derived from the patient's own blood.

Ayurveda is an Indian system of medicine that utilizes herbs, yoga, and other nontoxic techniques to bring the body into a state of harmony with the environment.

B.A. Bachelor of Arts.

B.Ac. Bachelor of Acupuncture.

Bach flower remedies are subtle essences originally refined in England. They are said to have powerful healing properties.

BCG (Bacillus Calmette-Guérin) is the tuberculosis vaccine that has been used in the treatment of cancer.

B.Ed. Bachelor of Education.

Beta-carotene is a derivative of vitamin A. It is widely accepted today as a cancer preventative.

Biofeedback is a technique based on the understanding that we can learn to regulate our own internal states, including that of the autonomic nervous system, which previously had been thought to be beyond our conscious control. Patients are hooked up to equipment that monitors their bodily functions and returns this information to the person in the form of visual, auditory, or tactile representations. It is said to be useful for controlling tension, migraine headaches, high blood pressure, anxiety, and insomnia. Through a series of sessions, the patient learns to trigger relaxation at will.

Biomagnetic and **micro frequencies**, according to some people, have the ability to destroy abnormal cells and harmful organisms, depending on the frequencies used.

Bovine cartilage is an immunostimulant used in treating cancer.

B.S. Bachelor of Science.

Butyrate complex is a combination of butyric acids. Its nontoxic fatty acids are used to stimulate interferon.

C.A. Certified Acupuncturist.

CAT scan (computerized axial tomography scanning) involves the passing of numerous X-rays through the brain to produce a composite three-dimensional picture.

Catabolic actions break down complex compounds, taken as food, into simpler compounds.

CBC (complete blood count) is a test that calculates the number of red and white cells per cubic millimeter of blood.

CEA (carcino-embryonic antigen) is a blood test used to determine the presence of cancerous cells.

Cell therapy, or cellular therapy, treats a dis-eased organ with the cells of a corresponding healthy organ. This consists of periodic injections of live or freeze-dried embryonic cells and tissues into the patient's muscular system. These injected cells are carried to the same type of cells within the body, where they work on the repair and revitalization of that tissue. Professor Niehans developed this method, which is popular in Europe. It is used to treat malignant diseases, diabetes, Down's syndrome, osteoporosis, central nervous system disorders, immune deficiency, impotence and sterility, and many other disorders. The embryonic cells used in the injections are usually removed from a healthy flock of black sheep.

Cesium chloride changes the pH of a cancer cell from acid to alkaline, making it difficult for the cell to reproduce and thereby slowing down growth, according to Dr. Keith Brewer. He says it does this without being toxic to normal cells.

Chelation therapy (EDTA): is a term derived from the Greek "chele," which means to claw or pick up. The solution contains EDTA (ethylene diamine tetracetic acid), which carries out heavy metals like lead, cadmium, and arsenic, as well as other foreign substances, many of which enter our bodies in our food, in the air, and in our water. Chelation is the process of surrounding or enclosing a mineral atom with a larger protein molecule. The purpose is to increase the flow of blood to the vital organs and tissues of the body by reducing calcium deposits in the arteries and blood vessels.

Chemotherapy is the treatment of disease with chemical agents.

Chondroitin sulfate, pioneered in Germany, consists of mucopolysaturates that stimulate blood flow.

Clinical ecology is a relatively new branch of medicine focusing on environmentally provoked illnesses. These illnesses often seem to occur in man-made environments.

C.M.D. Doctor, Master in Surgery.

C.N. Clinical Nutritionist.

C.N.C. Certified Nutritional Consultant.

Coenzyme Q$_{10}$ enhances body function by helping remove toxic foreign matter from the blood.

Coffee enemas are said to stimulate the liver to rid itself more effectively of deadly toxins. They were popularized in cancer treatment by Dr. Max Gerson and are used along with other cancer therapies as well. They must be prepared according to certain specifications.

Coley vaccine (toxins) incites a fever and is used in some cancer treatments.

Colonic irrigation is a gentle internal washing done by water under controlled pressure and temperature.

D.C. Doctor of Chiropractic.

D.D.S. Doctor of Dental Surgery.

D.H.M. Doctor of Homeopathic Medicine.

Diapulse treatment uses high-frequency electromagnetic energy to improve metabolism and general organ function.

D.M.D. Doctor of Dental Medicine.

DMSO (dimethyl sulfoxide) acts as an agent or vehicle that facilitates the penetration of anti-cancer drugs into the tumor.

D.N. Doctor of Naprapathy.

D.N.P. Doctor of Naturopathy.

D.O. Doctor of Osteopathy.

D.P. Doctor of Pharmacy.

D.P.M. Doctor of Podiatry.

D.Sc. Doctor of Science.

ECG (electrocardiogram) is a graphical record of cardiac function. The medical profession commonly refers to it as an EKG.

Ed.D. Doctor of Education.

EDTA. *See* Chelation therapy.

EKG. *See* ECG.

Essiac is an herbal concoction that has been widely used in Canada as a method of treating cancer. It is available through specific government approval of individual cases.

F.A.C.P. Fellow of the American College of Physicians.

F.C.A.P. Fellow of the College of American Pathologists.

Fever therapy, or pyretotherapy, has been found to be beneficial to the body in that lymphocytes will produce a great amount of antibodies when the body's temperature is high. These antibodies will destroy bacteria and toxins and help eliminate them, thus stimulating the immune system to work against the cancer. Fever is induced through the injection of a bacterial substance into the body.

Flutamide gets positive results with prostate cancer, according to discoveries by Dr. LaBrie in Canada.

Fred (fiche reticular endithelial differ-ential) tests were developed by Dr. Yves Augusti of France for determining the presence of cancer.

Germanium, a natural substance found in plants and foods, was found in Japan to be an oxygen enhancer, restoring to normal function the T-cells, the B-lymphocytes natural killer cell activity, and numbers of antibody-forming cells.

GH3, or Gerovital H3, was developed in Romania by Ana Aslan, M.D. It is used to treat a variety of degenerative conditions and to slow the aging process.

Hair analysis is painless, easy, and free of risks. A small amount of hair is taken from the nape of the neck to examine the intracellular (inside the cell) information of the person's condition for the last three months. This procedure reveals toxic metal levels and nutrient mineral levels.

H.D. Homeopathic Doctor.

Herbal therapy uses various herbal combinations for healing as well as cleansing purposes. These are used in the form of tablets, capsules, tinctures, extracts, and herbal baths with poultices. Herbs are a valuable adjunct to many therapies.

HLB (Hyton-Lygard Bradford) blood tests are used on patients to monitor the progress of their disease.

H.M.D. Holistic Medical Doctor; Homeopathic Doctor.

Homeopathy is a system of medicine based on the belief that the cure of disease can be effected by minute doses of substances that, if given to a healthy person in large doses, would produce the same symptoms as are present in the disease being treated. Homeopathy employs natural substances in small doses to stimulate the body's reactive process to remove toxic waste and bring the body back into balance. It was first used in the early 1800s by Samuel Hahnemann of Germany.

Hydrazine sulfate is an inexpensive chemical substance used to treat cachexia (wasting away). It is said to have anti-cancer properties.

Hydrogen peroxide, properly prepared and given orally or by infusion, is used to increase oxygen tension in the cancer cell. It is used for other degenerative diseases, too.

Hydrotherapy can include steam baths, whirlpools, foot baths, and mineral baths, all of which help remove toxins from the body, stimulate the entire nervous and muscular system, and increase circulation.

Hyperthermia is the artificial induction of exceptionally high fever for therapeutic purposes. Malignant cells cannot tolerate heat as well as normal cells can; therefore, the increased temperature destroys cancer cells and leaves normal cells intact. There are several ways of using hyperthermia, ranging from wet heat to dry heat.

Immunology is the science dealing with the specific mechanisms by which living tissues react to foreign biological material in a way that may enhance resistance or immunity. In mainstream medicine, such treatments include the use of monoclonal antibodies, interferon, interleukin-2, and TNF (tumor necrosis factor).

Immunotherapies are those therapies that strengthen the immune system. There is a wide range of therapies that are said to operate this way.

Interferon is a protein molecule that is created by white blood cells. It acts to keep viruses from multiplying.

Interleukins are hormone-like substances produced by lymphocytes. They often are used in mainstream biological therapies having strong side effects.

Iridology is the science of determining acute, sub-acute, chronic, and destructive stages in the affected organs of the body by examining their corresponding areas in the iris.

Iscador, or mistletoe, is an herb used mainly as an anti-cancer agent in anthroposophical medicine.

Jason Winters herbal tea is a combination of three herbs—red clover, chapparal, and an Oriental herb—that cured Jason Winters of his cancer.

Kirlian photography is a method of photographing objects by means of high-voltage spark discharges. The Kirlians describe their photography as a method for the conversion of properties of an object into electrical properties that are then captured on film.

Koch reagent (glyoxilide) is an oxidation catalyst used in very low dosage. It is believed to stimulate biochemical reactions that antagonize malignant cells. It is usually administered by injection into the muscle. The theory is that the anaerobic (non-oxidizing) metabolism of malignant cells may be part of the cause of malignancy, as well as an identifying characteristic of cancer cells. Stimulating oxidation results in an environment less favorable to cancer cells.

Laetrile (amygdalin) has been used as an anti-cancer agent. Although it is not a vitamin, this substance is also known as vitamin B_{17}. Drs. Ernest Krebs Jr. and Sr. did research with amygdalin. They found that it helped relieve pain and increase appetite, weight, and energy. Laetrile is used as a part of metabolic therapy that includes a special laetrile diet, and as part of an enzyme therapy that helps open the outer coat of the cancer cell. Then the cyanide in the laetrile and the body's own immune system are said to destroy the cancer cell. Benzaldahyde, another component, has been found to help in relieving pain.

M.A. Master of Arts.

M.Ac. Master of Acupuncture.

Macrobiotics is a lifestyle and diet adapted

from the Far East and made known in America by Michio Kushi. The principles of the diet consist of balancing the yin and yang energies of foods. In brief, yin foods, such as water, are expansive, while yang foods, such as salt or meat, are constrictive. For the most part, the diet consists of whole grain cereals, millet, rice, soups, and vegetable dishes, with beans and supplementary foods depending on the individual and the condition. Different types of cancers are considered either yin or yang, and the macrobiotic program must be adapted to each individual.

M.D. Doctor of Medicine.

Metabolic therapy usually consists of daily doses of amygdalin (laetrile), enzymes, and vitamin-mineral supplements. A diet is often recommended to complement this program. The diet centers on avoiding fats, salts, and sugars, and on eating plenty of raw vegetables and fruits.

M.H. Master Herbalist.

Monoclonal antibodies attack tumor antigens in specific cancers and are part of mainstream immunotherapy.

M.S. Master of Science.

M.Sc.D. Doctor of Medicinal Science.

M.S.N. Master of Science in Nursing.

M.S.W. Master of Social Work.

Naturopathy is a natural way of healing using many methods, including herbs, diet, osteopathy, hydrotherapy, sunlight, deep breathing, exercise, relaxation, and the removal of noxious influences.

N.D. Doctor of Naturopathy.

Noninvasive vascular testing is an electronic analysis of circulation. Changes in blood vessel walls in smokers and in patients suffering from diabetes, arteriosclerosis, and other causes of circulatory problems can be detected and analyzed.

Nuclear medicine is the branch of medicine that deals with the use of radioisotopes in diagnosis and therapy.

O.D. Doctor of Optometry.

O.M.D. Oriental Medicine Doctor.

Osteopathy is a school of healing that teaches that the body is a vital mechanical organism whose structural and functional integrity are coordinated and interdependent and that the abnormality of either constitutes disease. Its major contribution to treatment is manipulation.

Ozone that is designed for medical use is made by causing medically pure oxygen to flow over electrically charged surfaces. It is used mainly in three ways. One is to flow ozone gas over open lesions such as diabetic gangrene on feet, hands, arms, or legs. The ozone often eliminates any need for amputation of the extremity by destroying infections and promoting normal healing. Intravenous injections of ozone directly into the blood stream is another means of using ozone. The tiny bubbles formed when the ozone-oxygen is slowly injected through a fine needle are quickly dissolved into the blood stream. The third way is for ozone-oxygen to be introduced into the colon of adults. Ozone may help to destroy parasites and bacteria throughout the colon.

PABA (para-aminobenzoic acid) is a protective antioxidant vitamin used by the skin to filter out damaging ultraviolet radiation.

Pao D'Arco herbal tea, or lapochol or taheebo, is a South American tea made from tree bark generally found in Brazil or Argentina. The tea is said to have anti-cancer properties.

P.D. Doctor of Pharmacy.

pH is a measure of the acidity or alkalinity of a substance, using a scale from 0 (most acidic) to 14 (most alkaline), with 7 considered neutral.

Phar.G. Graduate in Pharmacy.

Phar.M. Master of Pharmacy.

Ph.C. Pharmaceutical Chemist.

Ph.D. Doctor of Philosophy.

Ph.T. Physical Therapist.

Plasmapheresis is employed as a therapeutic procedure in the treatment of several diseases. This procedure separates blood into its various components, isolating the plasma, red cells, white cells, and platelets in a continuous flow system. The typical plasmapheresis procedure involves separating the patient's red blood cells from the plasma. The red blood cells are then immediately returned to the patient, and the volume of plasma removed is replaced with fresh frozen plasma or with normal saline solution and albumin, which have properties similar to plasma. Plasmapheresis can also be used on some cancer patients, such as those whose tumors produce high quantities of abnormal proteins (e.g., multiple myeloma and related disorders). The plasmapheresis separates these proteins by removing the patient's plasma and replacing it with other compatible solutions.

P.M.D. Private Medical Doctor.

Polypeptides are compounds containing two or more amino acids united through the linkage of peptides, intermediates between the amino acids, and peptones in the synthesis of proteins.

Progenator cryptocides is a microbe, or bacterium, that is in the blood and can be seen through a darkfield microscope. According to Dr. Virginia Livingston, this microbe is the cause of cancer.

Proteolytic enzymes have a particular ability to break down certain proteins yet do not attack the beneficial proteins that make up the normal cells of the body. These enzymes are said to have great value in fighting cancer as well as many other diseases. If the body were always capable of producing adequate proteolytic enzymes, it is possible that cancer would not develop. In theory, cancer cells have a type of protein coating that is destroyed by proteolytic enzymes. When this protein is destroyed, the body's white cells are able to attack the cancer cells and destroy them.

Psychic surgery is peformed most frequently in the Philippines by psychic healers, who use only their hands to "remove" impurities from the patient's body. Reputedly, this surgery is quick and relatively painless. The healer closes up the "incision," no scar remains, and it takes very little time.

P.T. Physical Therapist.

Qi is the vital energy, or life force of tthe body, in traditional Chinese medicine.

Qi Gong, a Chinese form of yoga, is said to be very helpful in treating cancer. Its efficacy in the treatment of lung cancer is under investigation.

Radiation therapy is usually treatment with ionizing radiation, including Roentgen rays, radium, or other radioactive substances.

R.C.P. Respiratory Care Practitioner.

Rife microscope, developed by Dr. Royal Rife, enabled him to see harmful cells destroyed.

R.N. Registered Nurse.

Rolfing is a form of deep muscle body work developed by the late Dr. Ida Rolf.

R.P.T. Registered Physical Therapist.

714X is a camphor-based nontoxic substance that works against cancer, according to observations through a powerful microscope known as a Somatoscope. Gaston Naessens created both 714X and the Somatoscope.

Shark cartilage is an anti-cancer immuno-stimulant.

Shark liver extract, researched in Sweden as being helpful in leukemia cases, is now being used with other cancers, too.

Staphage-lysate is a microbial accumulation used to stimulate an immune response. It is sometimes called "the germ's germ."

Visualization is the use of mental imagery to create positive beliefs that will activate the body's defenses against disease. In visualization, images are perceived in the mind with such distinctness that they seem to be seen by the eyes.

Yoga (from the Sanskrit word for "union" or "oneness") is a personal self-help system of health care and spiritual development. Its founders were working in India about 2,000 years ago. This approach to becoming one with life involves meditation; postures or asanas, known as Hatha yoga; service to others, known as Karma yoga; devotion and love, known as Bhakti yoga; a vegetarian diet; and breathing methods that help calm the body and mind.

Bibliography

Because a great deal of literature has been written about alternatives in the field of cancer, the following list has been divided into six categories to help you find those books that are of greatest interest to you. Many, but not all, duplicate the Related Readings listed in the text. By no means does this bibliography include all of the books that have been written on this subject.

Books listed under "Comprehensive Overview" detail, to some degree, information about most alternative cancer therapies. Specific regimens can be found under "Program-Related Books." As far as possible, the regimen has been indicated whenever the title isn't self-explanatory. The "Survivor Stories" category includes firsthand accounts of patients' recoveries. In most cases, the therapy used has been indicated. Under "Mind: Behavioral-Psychological Aspects of Health," you will find many of the more important books in this growing area. "General Reading" is a kind of catchall for books that sometimes touch on one or more of the above subjects, and sometimes encompass much more. Additional regimens and programs, as well as books on the politics of cancer, can be found here. There is also a section of periodicals relating to cancer and alternative therapies.

If a book is not available through conventional sources and is still in print, try a center that is related to the subject matter, or contact the : Cancer Book House, 2043 North Berendo Street, Los Angeles, California 90027.

COMPREHENSIVE OVERVIEW

Alternative Medicine—The Definitive Guide—Breaking Through the Cancer Puzzle. Burton Goldberg. Future Medicine Publishing, 1997

Alternatives in Cancer Therapy—The Complete Guide to Non-Traditional Treatments. Ross Pelton, Ph.D. and Lee Overholser, Ph.D. Fireside, 1994.

The Cancer Solution. Robert E. Willner, M.D., Ph.D. Pelter Publishing, 1994.

Cancer Therapy—The Independent Consumer's Guide to Non-Toxic Treatment and Prevention. Ralph W. Moss, Ph.D. Equinox, 1992.

Choices in Healing—Integrating the Best of Conventional and Complementary Approaches to Cancer. Michael Lerner. MIT Press, 1994.

The Complete Guide to Alternative Cancer Therapies. Ron Falcone. Citadel Press, 1994.

Healing Your Body Naturally—Alternative Treatments to Illness. Gary Null. Four Walls, Eight Windows, 1992

Options—The Alternative Cancer Therapy Book. Richard Walters. Avery Publishing Group, 1992.

What Your Doctor Won't Tell You—The Complete Guide to the Latest in Alternative Medicine. Jane Heimlich. Harper Perennial, 1990.

When the Doctor Says It's Cancer. Robert L. Erdmann, Ph.D. Bioscience, 1994.

PROGRAM-RELATED BOOKS

Amygdalin (Laetrile) Therapy. Bruce W. Halstead, M.D. Choice Publications, Inc., 1977.

An Anthroposophical Approach to Cancer. Rita Leroi, M.D. Mercury Press, 1982.

Be Your Own Doctor: A Positive Guide to Natural Living. Ann Wigmore. Avery Publishing Group, 1982. (Wheatgrass and Raw Foods)

Biologically Closed Electric Circuits. Bjorn E.W. Nordenstrom. Stockholm: Nordic Medical Publications, 1983. (Altering Electrical Fields)

Bristol Programme. Penny Brohn. Century Hutchinson, 1987.

A Calling of an Angel. Dr. Gary L. Glum. Silent Walker Publishing, 1988. (Essiac)

The CanCell Controversy. Louise B. Trull. Hampton Roads Publishing Co., Inc., 1993.

Cancer: A Mandate to Humanity. Friedrich Lorenz. Mercury Press, Fellowship Community, 1982. (Anthroposophical Medicine)

Cancer: A New Breakthrough. Virginia Livingston-Wheeler, M.D. Livingston, 1972. (Livingston Treatment)

Cancer: A Second Opinion. Josef Issels, M.D. London: Hodder and Stoughton, 1975. (Issels Treatment)

Cancer and the Philosophy of the Far East. George Ohsawa. George Ohsawa Macrobiotic Foundation, 1981. (Macrobiotic Diet)

A Cancer Battle Plan. Anne E. Frähm with David J. Frähm. Piñon Press, 1992.

Cancer: Causes, Prevention and Treatment: The Total Approach. Paavo Airola. Health Plus Publishers, 1982. (Metabolic)

Cancer Holiday. Bettie Towner. Greenlake Publishers, 1978. (Discusses Several Clinics)

The Cancer Prevention Diet. Edward Esko, Editor. East West Foundation, 1981. (Macrobiotic Diet)

The Cancer Prevention Diet. Michio Kushi and Alex Jack. St. Martin's Press, 1983. (Macrobiotic Diet)

The Cancer Problem. Paul Niehans. Staempfli & Cie Ltd., 1969. (Cell Therapy)

Cancer Prophylaxis and Cancer Immunology. Paul Niehans. Staempfli & Cie Ltd., 1968. (Cell Therapy)

A Cancer Therapy: Results of 50 Cases. Max Gerson, M.D. Totality Books, 1977. (Gerson Therapy)

A Challenging Second Opinion. John A. McDougall, M.D. New Win, 1985.

Cleanse. Jason Winters. Vinton Publishing, 1984. (Jason Winters Program)

The Conquest of Cancer: Transcript From a Videotape Program. Virginia Livingston-Wheeler, M.D., and Owen Wheeler, M.D. (Livingston Treatment)

The Conquest of Cancer: Vaccines and Diet. Virginia Livingston-Wheeler, M.D., with Edmond G. Addeo. Franklin Watts Publishing, 1984. (Livingston Treatment)

The Cure for All Cancers. Hulda Regeher Clark, Ph.D., N.D. Promotion Publishing, 1993.

The Death of Cancer. Harold W. Manner. Advanced Century Publishing, 1978. (Manner Metabolic Protocol)

Diagnosis: Cancer—Prognosis: Life (the Story of Dr. Lawrence Burton). Jane Riddle Wright. Albright and Co., 1985. (Burton's Immuno-Augmentative Therapy)

Diet for Cancer. Virginia Livingston, M.D. (Livingston Treatment)

Dr. Kelley's Answer to Cancer. (Combines *One Answer to Cancer* by Kelley with *Metabolic Ecology* by Rohe.) Wedgestone Press, 1986.

Dr. Moerman's Anti-Cancer Diet. Ruth Jochems. Avery Publishing Group, 1990.

Dr. Nieper's Revolution. Hans Nieper, M.D. (Nieper Program)

An End to Cancer. Leon Chaitow, D.O. Wellingsborough, Northamptonshire, England: Thorens Publishers Ltd., 1985. (Dr. Chaitow's Program)

The Essiac Report. Richard Thomas. Atin, 1993.

The Famous Bristol Detox Diet. Alec Forbes, M.D. Keats Publishing, Inc. (Bristol Cancer Help Centre)

Galileo of the Microscope. Christopher Bird. Les Presses de l'Université de la Personne Inc., 1990. (Gaston Naessens)

A Gentle Way With Cancer. Brenda Kidman. London: Century Publishing, 1985. (Bristol Cancer Help Centre)

Gerson Therapy Handbook. Mary Lee Rork. 1981.

The Grape Cure. Johanna Brandt. Ehret Literature Publishing Co.

Homeopathic Medicine and Cancer. Robin Murphy. Homeopathic Research Project, National College of Naturopathic Medicine, 1979.

International Protocols IIMP in Cancer Management. Robert W. Bradford, et al. Robert W. Bradford Foundation, 1982. (American Biologics)

Killing Cancer: The Jason Winters Story. Jason Winters. England: Skilton and Shaw Publishing, 1980. (Jason Winters Herbal Tea)

Koch Remedy/Cancer. Borderland Sciences Research Foundation, 1986.

Laetrile: Case Histories. John A. Richardson, M.D., and Patricia Griffin. Bantam, 1977.

Laetrile/Control for Cancer. Glenn D. Kittler. Warner Paperback, 1973.

Little Cyanide Cookbook—B$_{17}$ Recipes. June de Spain. American Medic, 1978. (Laetrile Therapy)

The Macrobiotic Approach to Cancer. Michio Kushi. Avery Publishing Group, 1982.

The Macrobiotic Cancer Prevention Cookbook. Aveline Kushi with Wendy Esko. Avery Publishing Group, 1988.

A Matter of Life or Death: The Incredible Story of Krebiozen. Herbert Bailey. G.P. Putnam's Sons, 1958. (Krebiozen and Dr. Andrew Ivy)

Metabolic Cancer Therapies. Kurt W. Donsbach, M.D. International Institute of Natural Health Sciences, Inc., 1981.

Metabolic Cancer Therapy. Bruce W. Halstead, M.D. Golden Quill Publishers, Inc., 1978.

Metabolic Ecology: A Way to Win the Cancer War. Fred Rohe. Wedgestone Press, 1982. (Kelley Treatment)

The Metabolic Management of Cancer. Robert W. Bradford and Michael L. Culbert, Editors. Robert W. Bradford Foundation, 1979. (American Biologics)

Metabolic Therapy, A-1982 and C-1982. Dr. Harold W. Manner. Metabolic Research Foundation. (Manner Protocol)

The Microbiology of Cancer. Virginia Livingston-Wheeler, M.D. (Livingston Treatment)

The Natural Way to a Healthy Prostate. Michael Schacter, M.D. Keats Publishing, 1995.

The New Approach to Cancer. Cameron Stauth. English Brothers Press, 1982. (Kelley Treatment)

New Hope for Cancer Victims. William Donald Kelley, D.D.S. The Kelley Research Foundation, 1980. (Kelley Treatment)

Nutrition: The Cancer Answer. Maureen Salaman. Statford Publishing, 1983.

One Answer to Cancer. William Donald Kelley, D.D.S. Wedgestone Press, Kelley Research Foundation, 1974. (Kelley Treatment)

Raw Food Treatment Cancer/Other. Kristine Nolfi, M.D. Health Research.

Rejuvenation. Stephen Blauer. Green Gown Publications. (Raw Foods)

Research in Physiopathology as Basis of Guided Chemotherapy With Special Application to Cancer. Emanuel Revici, M.D. Van Nostrand, 1961. (Revici Treatments)

Revolution in Technology, Medicine and Society. Hans Nieper, M.D. Oldenburg: MIT Verlag, 1983. (Nieper)

Second Opinion: LaPacho and the Cancer Controversy. Bill Wead. Canada: Rostrom, 1985. (Pao D'Arco Herbal Tea)

Sharks Don't Get Cancer—How Shark Cartilage Could Save Your Life. Dr. I. William Lane and Linda Comac. Avery Publishing Group, 1992.

Sharks Still Don't Get Cancer. Dr. I. William Lane and Linda Comac. Avery Publishing Group, 1996.

Survival Into the 21st Century. Viktoras Kulvinskas. Omangod Press, 1975. (Wheatgrass and Raw Foods)

The Treatment of Cancer With Herbs. John Heinerman. BiWorld Publishers, 1980.

The Truth About Perisel. Jason Winters. M & R Publishers, 1982. (Jason Winters)

Why Suffer? Ann Wigmore. Avery Publishing Group, 1985. (Wheatgrass and Raw Foods)

The Yeast Connection. William Crook, M.D. Professional Books, 1986. (Anti-Candida)

You Don't Have to Die. Harry M. Hoxsey. Joseph C. Carl, 1977. (Hoxsey)

Your Own Perfect Medicine. Martha M. Christy. Futuremed, 1994. (Urine Therapy)

SURVIVOR STORIES

Beating the Odds. Albert Marchetti. Contemporary Books, 1988.

Cancer—One Man's Fight to Control Malignancy. Robert Stickle. Natural Foods Associates, 1976.

Cancer Support for the Surviving Soul. Jack Canfield, Mark Victor Hansen, Nancy Mitchell, R.N. Health Communications Inc., 1996.

Cancer Winner. Jaquie Davison. Pacific Press, 1977. (Gerson)

Confessions of a Kamikaze Cowboy. Dirk Benedict. Avery Publishing Group, 1991. (Macrobiotics)

Gentle Giants. Penny Brohn. London: Century Publishing. (Issels)

Health After Cancer—An Intelligent Approach to Recovery and True Health. Dale Figtree, Ph.D. Hanuman Press, 1985.

How I Conquered Cancer Naturally. Eydie Mae Hunsberger. Avery Publishing Group, 1992., (Wheat-grass and Raw Foods)

How I Healed My Cancer Holistically. Dore Deverell. Psychenutrition, Inc., 1978. (Kelley Treatment)

How I Overcame Inoperable Cancer. Wong Hon Sung. Exposition Press, 1975.

I Beat Cancer. Bernice Wallin. Contemporary Books, 1978. (BCG Vaccine)

I Fought Leukemia and Won. Rex B. Eyre. Hawkes Publishing, 1982. (Gerson)

Keep Your Breast: Preventing Breast Cancer the Natural Way. Susan Moss. Resource Publications, 1994.

My God, I Thought You'd Died. Claude Dosdall and Joanne Broatch. Bantam-Seal Books, 1986.

My Triumph Over Cancer. Beata Bishop. Keats Publishing, Inc., 1986. (Gerson)

A Rational Concept of Cancer. Robert Stickle. Natural Foods Associates, 1977.

Recalled by Life. Anthony Sattilaro, M.D. Avon Books, 1982. (Macrobiotics)

Thank God I Had Cancer. Rev. Clifford Oden. Cancer Book House, 1984.

Too Young to Die. Rick Hill. Hill Publications, 1979. (Contreras)

Vital Signs. Fitzhugh Mullan, M.D. Dell Publishing Co., Inc., 1983.

You Bet You Can. Tony Moscato, 1984. (Jason Winters Tea/Wheatgrass)

You Can Conquer Cancer. Ian Gawler. Australia: Hill of Content Publishing, 1985. (Gerson, Megavitamins, Psychic Surgery, Meditation)

MIND: BEHAVIORAL-PSYCHOLOGICAL ASPECTS OF HEALTH

Bridges of the Bodymind. Jeanne Achterberg and G. Frank Lawlis. Institute for Personality and Ability Testing, 1980.

Cancer as a Turning Point. Lawrence LeShan. Plume, 1990.

From Victim to Victor. Harold Benjamin, Ph.D. Dell, 1987.

Getting Well Again. O. Carl Simonton, M.D., Stephanie Matthews-Simonton, and James Creighton. J.P. Tarcher, 1978.

Healing and the Mind. Bill Moyers. Doubleday, 1993.

The Healing Family. Stephanie Matthews-Simonton. Bantam Books, 1984.

The Healing Mind. Irving Oyle. Celestial Arts, 1979.

Healing With Mind Power. Richard Shames, M.D. Rodale Press, 1978.

Healing With the Mind's Eye. Michael Samuels, M.D., with Nancy Samuels. Summitt, 1990.

The Human Patient. Naomi Remen, M.D. Anchor Press/Doubleday, 1980.

Hypnosis and Behavioral Medicine. Daniel P. Brown and Erika Fromm. Lawrence Erlbaum Associates Publishing, 1987.

Imagery in Healing: Shamanism and Modern Medicine. Jeanne Achterberg. Shambhala Publications, 1985.

Imagery of Cancer. Jeanne Achterberg and G. Frank Lawlis. Institute for Personality and Ability Testing, 1978.

Love Is Letting Go of Fear. Gerald G. Jampolsky, M.D. Celestial Arts, 1979.

Love, Medicine, and Miracles. Bernie S. Siegel, M.D. Harper Row Publishers, 1986.

Mind and Immunity: Behavioral Immunology. Steven E. Locke and Mady Hornig-Rohan. Institute for the Advancement of Health.

Mind Over Cancer. Colin Ryder Richardson. Great Britain: W. Foulsham Co., 1988.

Minding the Body, Mending the Mind. Joan Borysenko. Bantam New Age Books, 1988.

The Other Medicines. Richard Grossman. Doubleday, 1985.

Peace, Love, and Healing. Bernie S. Siegel, M.D. Harper Row, 1989.

The Psychobiology of Mind-Body Healing. Ernest Lawrence Rossi. W.W. Norton Co., Inc., 1986.

Psychological and Behavioral Treatments for Disorders Associated With the Immune System: An Annotated Bibliography. Steven E. Locke. Institute for the Advancement of Health.

Superimmunity. Paul Pearsall, Ph.D. Fawcett, 1987.

The Type C Connection—The Behavioral Links to Cancer and Your Health. Lydia Temoshok, Ph.D. and Henry Dreher. Random House, 1992.

You Can Fight for Your Life. Lawrence LeShan. M. Evans and Co., 1977.

You Can Heal Your Life. Louise Hay. Coleman, 1985.

GENERAL READING

AIDS, Cancer and the Medical Establishment. Raymond Keith Brown, M.D. Robert Speller Publishers, 1986.

Anatomy of an Illness. Norman Cousins. W.W. Norton and Co., 1979.

Beating Cancer With Nutrition. Dr. Patrick Quillin, M.D., and Noreen Quillin. Nutrition Times Press, 1994.

The Beneficial Effects of Bacterial Infections on Host Resistance to Cancer: End Results in 449 Cases. Helen Coley Nauts. Cancer Research Institute, Inc.

Beneficial Effects of Immunotherapy on Sarcoma of the Soft Tissues, Other Than Lymphosarcoma. Helen Coley Nauts. Cancer Research Institute, Inc.

Breast Cancer: A Nutritional Approach. Carlton Fredericks. Grosset & Dunlap, 1977.

Breast Cancer: Immunological Factors Affecting Incidence, Prognosis and Survival. Helen Coley Nauts. Cancer Research Institute, Inc.

Breast Cancer: What Your Doctor May Not Tell You About Prevention, Diagnosis, and Treatment. Steve Austin, N.D., and C. Hitchcock.

Breast Cancer? Breast Health! The Wise Woman Way. Susan S. Weed. Ash Tree Publishing, 1996.

Cancer: A Beginner's Guidebook of Hope. Jane Peters. Encouraging Words Publishing, 1991.

Cancer: A Healing Crisis. Jack Tropp. Exposition Press, 1980. (Gerson/Issels)

Cancer and Consciousness. Barry Bryant. Sigo Press, 1990.

Cancer and Its Nutritional Therapies. Richard Passwater. Keats Publishing, Inc., 1983.

Cancer and Natural Medicine. A Textbook of Basic and Clinical Research. John Boik. Oregon Medical Press, 1996.

Cancer and Nutrition. Charles B. Simone, M.D. Avery Publishing Group, 1992.

Cancer and Vitamin C. Ewan Cameron and Linus Pauling. Linus Pauling Institute of Science and Medicine, 1979.

The Cancer Biopathy. Wilhelm Reich. Farrar, Straus, and Giroux, 1973.

The Cancer Blackout. Maurice Natenberg. Cancer Book House, 1975.

The Cancer Blackout Amended. Nat Morris. Regent House, 1976.

Cancer Causes and Natural Controls. Lynn Dallin. Ashley Books, 1983.

The Cancer Connection. Larry Agran. St. Martin's Press, 1977.

The Cancer Conspiracy. Dr. Robert E. Netterberg and Robert T. Tailor. Pinnacle Books, 1981.

The Cancer Cure That Worked. Barry Lynes. Canada: Marcus Books, 1987.

Cancer, Disease of Civilization. Ebba Waerland. Provoker Press, 1980.

Cancer, Exercise, Wellness, and Rehabilitation. Eric P. Durak, MSc. M.H. & F., 1996.

The Cancer Industry: Unraveling the Politics. Ralph W. Moss. Paragon House, 1989.

Cancer, Metabolic Therapy, and Laetrile. Douglas Heinsohn, 1977.

Cancer: Myths and Realities of Cause and Cure. M.L. Kothari and L.A. Mehta. Marion Boyars, Inc., 1979.

Cancer 1985. Hellfried Sartori, M.D. Life Science Universal, 1984.

A Cancer Patient's Survival Manual. Barbara Huntington. Avant Publishing, 1983.

Cancer Prevention, Fallacies, and Some Reassuring Facts. Cyril Scott. England: Athene Publishing Co., Ltd., 1968.

The Cancer Survivors and How They Did It. Judith Glassman. Dial Press, 1983.

The Cancer Syndrome. Ralph W. Moss. Grove Press, 1980.

Cancer? Think Curable! The Gerson Therapy. S.J. Haught. Gerson Institute, 1983.

Cancer Treatment: Why So Many Failures? Richard Ericson. GE-PS Cancer Memorial, 1980.

The Complete Guide to Cancer Prevention. Henry Dreher. Harper and Row, 1988.

Confessions of a Medical Heretic. Robert Mendelsohn. Warner Books, 1980.

Coping With Cancer—How to Fight Cancer With Vitamins, Minerals, and Diet. John L. Sessions, D.O., and Morton Walker, D.P.M. Devin-Adair Publishers, 1985.

Coping With Prostate Cancer. Robert H. Phillips, Ph.D. Avery Publishing Group, 1994.

Coronary? Cancer? God's Answer: Prevent It! Richard Brennan. Harvest House, 1979.

Crackdown on Cancer With Good Nutrition. Ruth Yale Long. Nutrition Education Association, 1983.

Diet, Nutrition, and Cancer. Committee on Diet, Nutrition, and Cancer, Assembly of Life Sciences, National Research Council. National Academy Press, 1982.

Divided Legacy—A History of the Schism in Medical Thought (3 Vols.). Harris Livermore Coulter. North Atlantic Books, 1982.

Dr. Atkins' Health Revolution: How Complementary Medicine Can Extend Your Life. Bantam, 1990.

Dressed to Kill—The Link Between Breast Cancer and Bras. Sidney Ross Singer and Soma Grismaijer. Avery Publishing Group, 1995.

Everyday Cancer Risks and How to Avoid Them. Mary Kerney Levenstein. Avery Publishing Group, 1992.

Food Is Your Best Medicine. Henry G. Bieler, M.D. Vintage Books, 1973.

Food Pharmacy. Jean Carper. Bantam, 1988.

Foods That Heal. Maureen Salaman. Statford Press, 1989.

Foods That Heal. Dr. Bernard Jensen. Avery Publishing Group, 1988.

Formula for Life. Eberhard Kronhausen, Ed.D., and Phyllis Kronhausen, Ed.D., with Harry B. Demopoulos, M.D. 1989.

Free Radical—Albert St. Gyorgyi and the Battle Over Vitamin C. Ralph W. Moss. Paragon House, 1988.

Freedom From Cancer. Mike Culbert. 76 Press, 1976.

The Great Medical Monopoly Wars. P.J. Lisa. International Health Institute of Natural Health Sciences, 1986.

Green Barley Essence. Yoshihide Hagiwara, M.D. Keats Publishing, 1986.

The Healing of Cancer. Barry Lynes. Marcus Books, 1989.

Health and Healing. Andrew Weil, M.D. Houghton Mifflin Co., 1983.

Health Through God's Pharmacy. Maria Treben. Austria: Wilhelm Ennsthaler, 1984.

How to Prevent and Gain Remission From Cancer. John Tobe. Canada: Provoker Press, 1975.

The Immortal Cell—Why Cancer Research Fails. Dr. Gerald B. Dermer. Avery Publishing Group, 1994.

The Indispensable Cancer Handbook. Kathryn H. Salsbury and Eleanor Liebman Johnson. Wideview Books/PEI Books, Inc., 1981.

Integral Cancer Therapies. Michael Lerner. Commonweal, 1987.

Maria Treben's Cures. Maria Treben. Austria: Wilhelm Ennsthaler, 1986.

Meals That Heal. L. Anne Fransen. Nutritional Research and Development, 1985.

Medical Armageddon, Vols. I–IV. Michael Culbert. C and C Communications, 1994–1995.

Medical Dark Ages Circa 1984 or Cancer Alternative Therapies Cure Rates. Ralph Hovnanian. 1984.

Medical Nemesis. Ivan Illich. Bantam Books, 1976.

Medicine on Trial. Charles B. Inlander, Lowell S. Levin, and Ed Weiner. People's Medical Society, 1988.

Miracle Cure: Organic Germanium. Kazuhiko Asai, M.D. Harper Row, 1987.

Natural Health, Natural Medicine. Andrew Weil, M.D. Houghton Mifflin, 1990.

New Hope and Improved Treatments for Cancer Patients. David Holmes. England: Wentworth House.

New Hope for Cancer Victims. Richard Welch, M.D. Cancer Book House, 1965.

No More Cancer. Ruth Yale Long. Nutrition Education Association, Inc.

Now That You Have Cancer. Robert W. Bradford. Choice Publication, 1977. (American Biologics)

Osteogenic Sarcoma: End Results Following Immunotherapy With Bacterial Vaccines: 165 Cases or Following Bacterial Infections, Inflammation, or Fever: 41 Cases. Helen C. Nauts. Cancer Research Institute, Inc.

The Persecution and Trial of Gaston Naessens. Christopher Bird. H.J. Kramer, 1991.

The Politics of Cancer. Samuel S. Epstein, M.D. Anchor Press, Doubleday, 1979.

Prevention and Cure of Cancer. Mulhim A. Hassan, M.D. Exposition Press, 1983. (Focal Infection)

The Prime Cause and Prevention of Cancer. Otto Warburg. Cancer Book House, 1973.

Questioning Chemotherapy. Ralph W. Moss, Ph.D. Equinox Press, 1995.

Racketeering in Medicine—The Suppression of Alternatives. James Carter, M.D., Ph.D. Hampton Roads Publishing Co., Inc., 1991.

Recovery From Cancer. Elaine Nussbaum. Avery Publishing Group, 1992.

Repression and Reform in the Evaluation of Alternative Cancer Therapies. Robert G. Houston. IAT Patients' Association, 1988.

The Serpent on the Staff—The Unhealthy Politics of the Amercian Medical Association. Howard Wolinsky and Tom Brune. Jeremy P. Tarcher/Putnam, 1994.

Spontaneous Remission: An Annotated Bibliography. Brendan O'Regan and Caryle Hirshberg. Noetic Sciences, 1993.

The Stress of Life. Hans Selye, M.D. McGraw-Hill Book Co., 1978.

Survival Factor in Neoplastic and Viral Diseases. William Koch, M.D. Cancer Book House.

Tijuana Clinics. Sally Wolper. Promotion Publishing, 1995.

Tijuana Clinics—Questions and Answers. Sally Wolper. Wolper Publications, 1983.

The Topic of Cancer. Dick Richards, M.D. England: Pergamon Press, 1982.

Unhealthy Charities—Hazardous to Your Health and Wealth. James T. Bennett and Thomas J. DiLorenzo. Basic Books, 1994.

Vitamin C Against Cancer. H.L. Newbold, M.D. Stein & Day Publishers, 1979.

Vitamins Against Cancer. Kedar N. Prasad. Nutrition Publishing House, Inc., 1989.

Winning the Fight Against Breast Cancer: The Nutritional Approach. Carlton Fredericks. Grosset Dunlap, 1979.

World Without Cancer: The Story of Vitamin B$_{17}$. G. Edward Griffin. American Media, 1980.

You Can Prevent Breast Cancer! Harvey Diamond. Promotion Publishing, 1995.

PERIODICALS

Alternative Medicine Digest. 1640 Tiberon Boulevard, Suite 2, Tiberon, CA 94920. (800) 333-HEAL.

Alternative Therapies. 101 Columbia, Aliso Viejo, CA 92656. (800) 899-1712.

Alternatives for the Health-Conscious Individual. Mountain Home Publishing, P.O. Box 829, Ingram, TX 78025. (210) 367-4492.

The Cancer Chronicles. c/o Equinox Press, 144 St. John's Place, Brooklyn, NY 11217.

The Choice. 1180 Walnut Avenue, Chula Vista, CA 91911. (619) 429-8200.

Explore for the Professional and *Explore More: Choices for a Better World.* P.O. Box 1508, Mount Vernon, WA 98273. (360) 424-6034/ (360)424-6025. Fax: (360) 424-6029.

The Gerson Healing Newsletter. P.O. Box 430, Bonita, CA 91908-0430.

Health Freedom News. P.O. Box 688, Monrovia, CA 91017. (818) 357-2181.

Hippocrates News. 1443 Palmdale Court, W. Palm Beach, FL 33411. (407) 471-8876.

Natural Health. 17 Station Street, Box 1200, Brookline Village, MA 02147. (800) 526-8440.

Options. P.O. Box 10, Otho, Iowa 50569. (515) 972-4444.

Townsend Letter for Doctors and Patients. 911 Tyler Street, Port Townsend, WA 98368. (360) 385-6021. Fax: (360) 385-0699.

The Wellness Network. 7807 Artesian Road, San Diego, CA 92127-2117. (619) 759-2966.

World Research News. 15300 Ventura Boulevard, Suite 405, Sherman Oaks, CA 91403. (818) 907-5483.

QUESTIONNAIRE FOR PATIENTS

It would be extremely helpful if we were able to get some information regarding your experiences with therapies, education programs, support groups, and information organizations. Any information will be confidential if requested, and can be submitted without a name if desired. Such information could be an invaluable service to people like you searching for assistance. Please return the completed questionnaire to the following address: Third Opinion, P.O. Box 50114, Santa Barbara, California 93150.

Name: _____

Address: _____

_____

_____

Patient's Name (if different from above): _____

Name of center, program, or service: _____

_____

Location: _____

_____

_____

Attending physician/health care provider: _____

Diagnosis: _____

_____

_____

_____

Treatment: _____

_____

_____

_____

_____

_____

_____

_____

_____

Effectiveness: _____
_____
_____
_____
_____

Length of stay: _____
_____
_____

Cost: _____
_____

Difficulties encountered (if any): _____
_____
_____
_____
_____
_____

Results: _____
_____
_____
_____
_____
_____

Comments: _____
_____
_____
_____
_____
_____
_____
_____

Index